Herbs That Heal
Natural Remedies for Good Health

The Magic: Herbs act in almost magical and astonishing ways—spasms may relax, pains vanish, constipation overcome, nervousness recede, headaches disappear, colds be banished, allergies counteracted, fevers controlled, blood flow arrested...the magic is endless.

The Heritage: Since early Neanderthal man, plants and herbs have been used for healing purposes and maintaining good health. Even as medical science has progressed, methods and ideas based on herbal healing have sustained and grown in different countries, across different cultures, often being used in exactly the same way. Bitter chamomile, for instance, is used as digestive aid throughout the world.

The Proof: Traditional herbal remedies have led scientists to the development of numerous 'modern' drugs; from aspirin, tranquilizers and *chywanprash* to heart saving digitalis, establishing beyond doubt the efficacy of 'herbal medicine'.

The Book: The book covers more than one hundred herbs, most of which are readily available (some even in your kitchen) or easily obtainable, and describes their specific healing properties, how the herb is useful in alleviating or preventing specific ailments; in most cases, the method of making and using herbal preperations is also explained. Index of ailments which can be treated by herbs makes the book specially useful.

The Author

H.K. Bakhru enjoys a countrywide reputation as an expert naturopath and a writer on the subject. His well-researched articles on nature cure, health, and nutrition appear regularly in the media.

He began his career in the Indian Railways with a first class first postgraduate degree from Lucknow University. He retired, in 1984, as the Chief Public Relations Officer of the Central Railways, after 35 years of distinguished service in the Public Relations Organisation of the Indian Railways and the Railway Board.

A diploma holder in Naturopathy, he is a member of the Nature Cure Practitioners' Guild in Bombay. He has made extensive studies on naturopathy and herbalism. He spends his retired life propagating and practising nature cure and is always willing to offer advice to those who seek his help. His other books on nature cure and nutrition are, *Foods That Heal, Vitamins That Heal, Natural Home Remedies for Common Ailments, Health the Natural Way, Diet Cure for Common Ailments, A Handbook of Natural Beauty, Nature Cure for Children's Diseases, Natural Health for the Elderly,* and *A Complete Handbook of Nature Cure.* He can be contacted at B-23, Hari Niwas, New Bombay Railwaymen's Cooperative Housing Society, Sector-2, Vashi, Navi Mumbai-400 703, Tel: 782 5967, Fax: 782 6239.

HERBS
THAT HEAL
Natural Remedies For Good Health

H.K. Bakhru

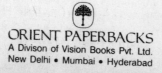

ORIENT PAPERBACKS
A Divison of Vision Books Pvt. Ltd.
New Delhi • Mumbai • Hyderabad

ISBN 81-222-0133-4

1st Published 1990
10th Printing 1998
11th Printing 1998
12th Printing 1999

Herbs That Heal: Natural Remedies for Good Health

© H.K. Bakhru

Cover design by Vision Studio

Published by
Orient Paperbacks
(A division of Vision Books Pvt. Ltd.)
Madarsa Road, Kashmere Gate, Delhi-110 006

Printed in India at
Kay Kay Printers, Delhi-110 007

Cover Printed at
Ravindra Printing Press, Delhi-110 006

Preface

Botanically, a herb is a plant with a non-woody stem which withers and dies down after flowering. In common usage, however, the term applies to all plants whose leaves, stems, roots, flowers, fruits or seeds have culinary or medicinal uses. This criterion forms the basis of the herbs included in this book.

This book is written as a companion volume to *Foods That Heal: The Natural Way to Good Health,* first published in 1990, reprinted twice in 1991 and again in 1992. The plants mentioned in the earlier book have therefore been omitted in this book though many of them qualify as 'herbs'. Exceptions have, however, been made in case of bael, fenugreek, garlic, ginger, Indian gooseberry and onion, as no book on herbs can be complete without the mention of these herbs due to their exceptional medicinal virtues.

The book covers 107 herbs and their medicinal uses in the treatment of diseases. It is divided into two parts. The first part describes, in some detail, 66 important herbs with strong healing power and curative properties; the second part describes, in brief, 41 herbs with comparatively milder properties. In each part herbs have been arranged alphabetically, according to their English names in most cases, and by trade name in a few cases, where they are more popular by trade names than their English names.

While there are numerous books on herbs, the distinctive feature of this book is its reasonably comprehensive information about herbs, especially their uses in the treatment of various diseases, at a reasonable price, for a wide readership.

H.K. Bakhru

Contents

Preface / 5
**Index of Diseases Which Responds
to Herbal Treatment / 9**
Introduction / 17

PART - I
H E R B S
Healing Power and Curative Properties

The popular Indian names are given in italics.

PART - II

M O R E H E R B S

Healing Power and Curative Properties

Index of Diseases and Ailments

An alphabetical list/index of diseases, common ailments which respond to healing power and curative properties of herbs.

Abdominal Pains
    See under Chronic Peritonitis

Acidity
    See under Indigestion

Acne
    See under Pimples

Anaemia
    Ash Gourd
    Celery
    Chicory
    Dill
    Fenugreek
    Gokulakanta
    Hog Weed
    Onion
    Wormwood

Arthritis/Rheumatism
    Alfalfa
    Blood Wort
    Castor Seeds
    Celery
    Chirayata
    Colchium
    Ephedra
    Garlic
    Gokulakanta
    Indian Aloe
    Indian Gooseberry
    Indian Sarsaparilla
    Indian Senna
    Indian Squill

Ispaghula
Leadwort
Lemon Grass
Madhuca
Nutmeg
Pepper
Rosemary
Saffron
Sage
Turpeth
Vasaka
Winter Cherry

Asthma/Bronchitis
    Aniseed
    Arjuna
    Asafoetida
    Bay Berry
    Bishop's Weed
    Black Nightshade
    Calamus
    Celery
    Chebulic Myroblan
    Chicory
    Clove
    Datura
    Ephedra
    Euphorbia
    Garlic
    Ginger
    Hermal
    Hog Weed
    Holy Basil

Hyssop
Indian Acalypha
Indian Gooseberry
Indian Squill
Kantakari
Linseed
Marjoram
Pergularia
Rhubarb
Rough Chaff
Saussurea
Turmeric
Vasaka

Burns, Scalds & Boils
Betel Leaves
Butea
Chalmogra
Chebulic Myroblan
Cumin Seeds
Curry Leaves
Dill
Indian Mallow
Madhuca
Margosa
Marigold
Parsley
Tamarind
Turmeric
Winter Cherry
Zizyphus

Cataract
Aniseed
Fenugreek
Garlic
Indian Mallow
Indian Sorrel
Parsley

Catarrah
Aniseed

Cholera
Clove
Fenugreek

Indian Barberry
Lemon Grass
Margosa
Onion
Poppy Seeds
Rough Chaff

Chronic Peritonitis/Colic/ Abdominal Pains
Bishop's Weed
Bitter Chamomile
Blood Wort
Cassia
Coriander
Cumin Seeds
Dill
Ginger
Hog Weed
Indian Spikenard
Ispaghula
Marjoram
Saffron
Zizyphus

Cirrhosis of Liver
See under Liver Problems

Common Cold
Bishop's Weed
Cassia
Cinnamon
Cumin Seeds
Ginger
Holy Basil
Hyssop
Nutmeg
Onion
Pepper
Vasaka

Conjuctivitis/Opthalmia
Babul
Coriander
East Indian Rosebay
Hog Weed
Indian Barberry

Marigold
Parsley
Pergularia
Rough Chaff
Tenner's Casia

Constipation
Bael Fruit
Belleric Myroblan
Betel Leaves
Cassia
Chebulic Myroblan
Chicory
Cinnamon
Fennel
Hog Weed
Indian Aloe
Indian Podophilla
Indian Senna
Ispaghula
Linseed
Liquorice
Parslane
Peepal
Picrorhiza
Rhubarb
Snake Gourd
Tamarind

Corns
Indian Squill
Marigold
Liquorice

Cough/Sore Throat
Bay Berry
Belleric Myroblan
Betel Leaves
Butea
Cardamon
Clove
Euphorbia
Fennel
Fenugreek
Garlic

Ginger
Henna
Hog Weed
Holy Basil
Indian Aloe
Linseed
Liquorice
Madhuca
Pepper
Rough Chaff
Sage
Tenner's Casia
Turmeric
Vasaka

Dandruff
See under Falling Hair

Dengue Fever
See under Fever

Depression
Cardamon

Dhobi's Itch
See under Ringworm

Diabetes
Butea
Curry Leaves
Fenugreek
Indian Gooseberry
Madhuca
Tenner's Casia

Diarrhoea & Dysentery
Arjuna
Babul
Bael Fruit
Banyan
Belleric Myroblan
Bishop's Weed
Black Nightshade
Butea
Chebulic Myroblan
Chicory
Cumin Seeds

Curry Leaves
Dill
Fenugreek
Henna
Holy Basil
Indian Gooseberry
Indian Pennywort

Diptheria
Garlic

Dropsy
Alfalfa
Arjuna
Belleric Myroblan
Black Nightshade
Digitalis
Euphorbia
Gokulakanta
Kantakari
Marjoram
Rough Chaff

Dysentery
See under Diarrhoea

Dyspepsia
See under Indigestion

Dysuria
Kantakari
Parslane
Sandalwood

Earache
Bael Fruit
Bishop's Weed
Bitter Chamomile
Clove
Ginger
Holy Basil

Eczema
Babul
Butea
Linseed
Madhuca

Falling Hair & Dandruff
Alfalfa
Ash Gourd
Curry Leaves
Euphorbia
Fenugreek
Indian Hemp
Rosemary
Sage
Trailing Eclipta

Fever/Dengue Fever
Bloodwort
Cassia
Chirayata
Coriander
Datura
Devil's Tree
Ephedra
Fenugreek
Hermal
Hog Weed
Holy Basil
Indian Bay Berry
Indian Mallow
Indian Sorrel
Lemon Balm
Lamon Grass
Pergularia
Saffron
Sandalwood
Snake Gourd
Tenner's Casia

Flatulence
See under Indigestion

Gall Stones
Celery
Kantakari

Glaucoma
Indian Gooseberry

Gout
Castor Seeds

Celery
Gokulkanta
Holy Basil
Turpeth
Zizyphus

Glycosuria
Asoka
Bay Berry
Butea
Calamus
Chirayata
Devil's Tree
Ispaghula
Indian Barberry
Indian Sarsaparilla
Jaundice Berry
Leadwort
Nutmeg
Parslane
Peepal
Pergularia
Poppy Seeds
Rhubarb
Rough Chaff
Sandalwood
Vasaka
Wood Apple

Headaches & Migraine
Betel Leaves
Bishop's Weed
Clove
Ginger
Henna
Indian Hemp

Heart Disorders
Alfalfa
Arjuna
Blood Wort
Digitalis
Garlic
Hog Weed
Indian Gooseberry
Kantakari

Lemon Balm
Onion
Peepal
Snake Gourd

Herpes
Linseed

High Blood Pressure
Alfalfa
Bloodwort
Garlic
Jaundice Berry
Parsley
Rauwolfia

Hysteria
Asafoetida
Ash Gourd
Picrorhiza
Rauwolfia
Saffron
Turmeric

Indigestion/Dyspepsia/Flatulence/Acidity
Aniseed
Belleric Myroblan
Bishop's Weed
Bitter Chamomile
Bloodwort
Calamus
Caraway Seeds
Cardamom
Cassia
Celery
Cheublic Myroblan
Cinnamon
Clove
Coriander
Cumin Seeds
Curry Leaves
Devil's Tree
Dill
Ephedra
Fennel

Fenugreek
Ginger
Hyssop
Indian Aloe
Indian Sarsaparilla
Indian Spikenard
Jaundice Berry
Lemon Grass
Marjoram
Margosa
Pepper
Picrorhiza
Rosemary
Saffron
Saussurea
Tamarind
Turmeric

Influenza
Fenugreek
Holy Basil
Marjoram
Onion
Zizyphus

Insomnia
Aniseed
Celery
Cumin Seeds
Indian Hemp
Indian Sorrel
Nutmeg
Poppy Seeds
Rauwolfia
Valerian

Intestinal Worms
Ash Gourd
Bamboo
Belleric Myroblan
Butea
Chirayta
East Indian Rosebay
Indian Acalypha
Indian Aloe
Indian Senna

Parslane
Snake Gourd
Turmeric
Wormwood

Jaundice
Chicory
Gokulakanta
Hog Weed
Indian Aloe
Indian Pennywort
Jaundice Berry
Parsley
Picrorhiza
Snake Gourd

Kibes
Banyan

Kidney Stones
Celery
Holy Basil

Leucoderma
Garlic
Holy Basil
Leadwort

Leucorrhoea
Asafoetida
Asoka
Babul
Banyan
Butea
Henna

Liver Problems & Cirrhosis of Liver
Chicory
Dandelion
Garlic
Henna
Hog Weed
Indian Aloe
Jaundice Berry
Kantakari
Lemon Balm

Picorrhiza
Snake Gourd

Low Blood Pressure
Indian Spikenard
Rauwolfia

Low Back Pain/Lumbago
Betel Leaves
Garlic
Indian Aloe
Lemon Grass
Rhubarb
Saffron

Lumbago
See under Low
Back Pain

Measles
Cinnamon
Turmeric

Menstrual Problems
Asafoetida
Asoka
Bamboo
Blood Wort
Chicory
Dill
Ginger
Henna
Hermal
Indian Hemp
Indian Spikenard
Indian Squill
Jaundice Berry
Lemon Grass
Pergularia
Tenner's Casia

Muscular Cramps
Clove
Ginger
Kantakari
Liquorice
Pepper

Myopia
Liquorice

Nausea
Cassia
Carry Leaves
Hog Weed

Nephritis
Linseed
Parsley

Opthalmia
See under Conjuctivitis

Orchitis
Madhuca

Peptic Ulcer
Ash Gourd
Bael Fruit

Pharyngitis
Cardamom

Pimples/Acne
Arjuna
Cinnamon
Coriander
Fenugreek
Sandalwood

Pleurisy
Celery
Hog Weed
Linseed

Prickly Heat
Sandalwood

Psoriasis
Black Nightshade

Pyorrhoea
Holy Basil
Pepper

Rheumatism
See under Arthritis

Ringworm/Dhobi's Itch
Butea
Cassia
Coriander
Cumin Seeds
Holy Basil
Hyssop
Indian Squill
Leadwort
Lemon Grass
Turmeric

Scalds
See under Burns

Sciatica
Bitter Chamomile
Indian Aloe
Nutmeg

Scurvy
Jaundice Berry
Wood Apple

Sinusitis
Ephedra
Fenugreek

Sore Throat
See under Cough

Sprain
Hyssop
Marjoram
Turmeric

Syphillis
Gokulakanta
Indian Mallow
Indian Pennywort
Poppy Seeds

Tonsilitis
Babul
Kantakari
Madhuca

Toothache/Teeth Disorders
Asafoetida

Babul
Banyan
Bay Berry
Clove
East Indian Rosebay
Holy Basil
Indian Mallow
Marjoram
Onion
Pepper

Teeth Disorders
See under Toothache

Tuberculosis
Ash Gourd
Celery
Chalmogra
Ginger
Indian Hemp
Linseed
Marigold
Onion
Winter Cherry

Typhoid
Jaundice Berry

Ulcer
Bamboo
Fenugreek
Hog Weed
Leadwort
Marigold
Parslane

Vaginitis
Chebulic Myroblan

Whitlow
Chebulic Myroblan
Ispaghula

Whooping Cough
Datura
Garlic

Introduction

The practice of herbal medicine dates back to the very earliest periods of known human history. There is evidence of herbs having been used in the treatment of diseases and for revitalising body systems in almost all ancient civilizations—the Indian, the Egyptian, the Chinese and even the Greek and Roman civilizations. Plants were the mainstay of medicine and credited with mystical and almost supernatural powers of healing. So much so that in Britain herbs became a focus of superstition, reaching their peak of importance in the Middle Ages when every village had its witch, and every witch her herbs and potions. Herbs were also used to counteract the witches' powers. Garlic, hyssop and wormwood all combated witchcraft and evil spirits.

In India, the records indicate, that herbs have been in use for treating diseases since ancient times. There are references to the curative properties of some herbs in the *Rigveda*, which is believed to have been written between 3500 and 1800 BC. Many of the plants mentioned in the *Rigveda* can be identified with reasonable certainty, although references to plants in *Rigveda* are very sketchy. A more detailed account is found in the *Atharvaveda*. A fairly comprehensive information about herbs has been recorded in *Charaka Samhita* and *Shusruta Samhita*—the two most important works on Ayurvedic system of medicine. The latter deals with as many as 700 herbs, some of which have not even originated in India. In subsequent years, more and more plants were used in indigenous medicine and their number gradually increased to 1500. The Chinese also have a compilation of 1,000 ancient herbs. *Pen Ts'ao Ching* is an important ancient Chinese work dating back to 2800 BC approximately, which describes various plant medicaments and instructions on their use. Hippocrates (460 BC),

17

the Greek physician and father of modern medicine also listed several hundred herbal remedies.

In recent years, researchers like O.C. Dutt, G. Watt, R.N. Chopra, K.R. Kirtikar, B.D. Basu, B. Mukherjee, the editors of *Wealth of India* and many others who have interest in plants and herbs, have done laborious and commendable work in compiling details of Indian medicinal plants. The studies conducted by these scholars have confirmed many of the claims of ancient herbalists about the efficacy of several herbs in curing diseases.

Herbs play a significant role, specially in modern times, when the damaging effects of food processing and over-medication have assumed alarming proportions. They are now being increasingly used in cosmetics, foods and teas, as well as alternative medicines. The growing interest in herbs is a part of the movement towards change in life-styles. This movement is based on the belief that the plants have a vast potential for their use as a curative medicine.

Herbs are used in many different ways. However, the ultimate objective of their use is that they should interact directly with our body chemistry. They may be used in various forms like food, medicine, cosmetics, or fragrance, but in all cases, their active constituents must be absorbed into the body for deriving the required benefits. Once they are absorbed in the bloodstream, they circulate to influence our whole system. The skill of the herbalist is to use this effect to balance and strengthen the body's own healing mechanism instead of suppressing or disturbing it, as many modern drugs tend to do.

The active constituents of the herb can enter the body in several ways. These include consuming the herb orally so as to be absorbed by the digestive system, application on skin through medicinal poultices as well as cosmetics for being absorbed in the body through the pores; application on eyes through lotions and compresses; smelling the aroma through nose to enable the essential oil being absorbed in the bloodstream.

Finally, a word of caution. While most herbs have little or no harmful side effects, some herbs may cause slightly undesirable reactions in some persons. Therefore, try only one herb at a time, beginning in small doses and wait and watch for side effects. If there are none, increase the use or dosage cautiously. Also, not all herbal applications are effective in every case in every person. And in no case should these be used as substitutes for professional medical attention in emergencies or serious chronic diseases.

18

PART 1

Alfalfa

Botanical Name: *Medicago satina*
Indian Name: *Alfalfa*

Origin, Distribution and Composition

Alfalfa is nutritionally one of the most versatile herbs yet discovered. It is a leguminous herb which grows upto 50 cms in height. It has rich green alternate leaves, purplish flowers and adapts itself to widely varying conditions of soil and climate.

Alfalfa appears to have been discovered by the Arabs who called it the "king of kings" of plants and the "father of all foods". They have used it for centuries to feed thoroughbred horses. The Persians recognized it as a healing grass.

Alfalfa is a native of Europe. It is now widely cultivated in the temperate regions, the subtropics and at higher altitudes in the tropics. It is grown throughout India.

Alfalfa is a valuable source of vitamins A,B,D,E and G. It also has some vitamin C and K. The rich quality, quantity and proper balance of calcium, magnesium, phosphorus, chlorine, sodium, potassium and silicon is of special value in alfalfa. All these elements are needed for the proper functioning of the various organs in the body.

Investigations made by the US Department of Agriculture have revealed that alfalfa contains one and a half times more protein than grains like wheat and corn and that its carbohydrate content is only half of that found in grains. The alfalfa proteins contain essential amino acids such as arginine, lysine, theronine and tryptophane. These amino acids supplement any deficiencies due to lack of essential nutrients in the diet.

Alfalfa is one of the richest sources of dietary fibre and chlorophyl. These nutrients have induced nutritional authorities to experiment with alfalfa as a ready form of easily digestible food and as a protein concentrate for supplementing protein-deficient foods such as vegetables.

Healing Power and Curative Properties

The seeds, leaves and stems of the alfalfa plant have important properties—derived from the roots of the plant which reach upto 12 metres into the subsoil and absorb the elusive trace minerals from the depths. The most important of these trace

21

minerals is manganese, which is vital to the human digestive system in its manufacture of insulin.

Alfalfa is an outstanding alkalizing food. It contains 130 to 142 mg of alkali-forming elements in every 100 grams.[1] These make it a valuable remedy for several ailments. It is slightly laxative, digestive, diuretic and serves as an excellent tonic. It augments the peristalsis or movement of the bowels, improves digestion and ensures better assimilation of food. Alfalfa builds up for a healthy and vigorous old age and resistance to infection.

Dropsy

An effective diuretic, alfalfa acts gently upon the kidneys. It can be successfully employed in the treatment of the inflammation of the bladder and dropsy, a disease marked by accumulation of fluid in the body.

Heart Disorders

Alfalfa, in the form of juice, has been found very effective in most arterial problems and heart diseases. Only fresh leaves of the plant may be used for this purpose. The juice of fresh alfalfa, however, is strong and potent and is best taken with carrot juice. In this combination, the individual benefits of each juice are intensified.

Respiratory Disorders

Alfalfa juice, as a rich source of chlorophyl, is useful in respiratory disorders and discomforts, particularly those relating to the sinuses and the lungs.

Stomach Disorders

The seeds of alfalfa, known as "king of sprouts", are of immense value in the maintenance of health. Their daily use helps build up an immunity to stomach distress. Alfalfa, in the form of tea, provides vital alkalizing benefits for hyperacidity. It tends to control the flow of hydrochloric acid, aiding the action of the gastric enzyme, pepsin. The addition of mint to alfalfa tea helps settle disturbed stomachs after a rich meal. It also refreshes the palate and makes an excellent morning drink.

---

1. Dr. S.J. Singh, *Food Remedies,* 4th edition, p.10, Nature Cure Council of Medical Research, Lucknow.

Arthritis

Alfalfa tea, especially made from the seeds, is of great value in arthritis, as it helps alkalize the food residues in the body. Six or seven cups of it should be taken daily by arthritics for at least two weeks.

Hair Disorders

The juice of alfalfa in combination with those of carrot and lettuce, if taken daily, helps the growth of hair to a remarkable extent. Such combination of juices is rich in elements which are beneficial for the roots of the hair.

High Blood Pressure

The herb is an effective remedy for high blood pressure. It contains all the elements necessary for the softening of hardened arteries, which characterise high blood pressure.

Methods for Uses: Alfalfa is used in many ways or forms. The seeds are useful in the form of sprouts. They are delicious and nourishing in salads and soups as well as in sandwiches. Alfalfa can be used in the form of juice extracted from its leaves. It is also used extensively in the form of tea, which is made from seeds as well as the dried leaves of the plant. The tea is prepared by boiling alfalfa seeds in an enamel pan with the lid on, for half an hour. It is strained, squeezing or pressing the seeds dry, and allowed to cool. Cold or hot water and honey maybe added to taste before use.

Aniseed

Botanical Name: *Pimpinella anisum*
Indian Name: *Velaiti saunf*

Origin, Distribution and Composition

Anise is an annual culinary herb belonging to *ajwain* or celery family. Its fruit, known as aniseed, is one of the oldest spices. The seed is ground-grey to greyish-brown in colour, oval in shape and 3.2 to 4.8 mm in length. It has an agreeable odour and a pleasant taste. The anise plant grows upto a height of 75 cms. It requires sunshine and warmth and does not grow satisfactorily in the tropical lowlands.

Anise is a native of the Middle East. It was cultivated by the ancient Egyptians, who valued its medicinal properties and culinary uses. It was also known to the early Greeks and Romans. It is now cultivated in Europe, Asia Minor, India and Mexico.

It contains moisture, substantial amount of protein, fatty oil and crude fibre besides essential oil, sugars, starch and ash. It also contains choline.

Anise oil is a colourless or pale-yellow liquid, with the characteristic odour and taste of the fruit. This oil has now replaced the fruits for medicinal and flavouring purposes.

The chief constituent of anise oil is anethole which is present in large quantity and is mainly responsible for the characteristic flavour of the oil. The oil also contains methyl, chavicol, p-methoxyphenyl acetone and small amounts of terpenes and sulphur compounds of disagreeable odour.

Healing Power and Curative Properties

Aniseed is esteemed in medicine for its properties to relieve flatulence and to remove catarrhal matter and phelgm from the bronchial tube. These properties are due to the presence of its essential oil. The seed also induces copious perspiration and increases the volume and discharge of urine.

Digestive Disorders

Aniseed is an ideal medicine for expelling wind from the stomach. It can also be taken, in combination with other digestives like ginger, cummin and pepper, in the form of an infusion. Gripe water for infants contains aniseed extract.

An easy way to prepare the infusion is to mix a teaspoon of aniseed in a cup of boiling water and leave it covered overnight. The clear fluid is then decanted and taken with honey. This is an ideal treatment for indigestion, especially when there is gurgling in the abdomen. It is also useful in preventing gas and fermentation in the stomach and the bowels.

Cataract

The herb is useful in the treatment of cataract. In such case, 6 grams of aniseed should be taken daily in the morning and evening. The other way of taking this herb is to powder an equal weight of aniseed and coriander seeds and to mix it with an equal weight of unrefined sugar. About 12 gram doses of this mixture is to be taken in the morning and evening.

Asthma

Aniseed is considered beneficial in the treatment of asthma due to its expectorant properties.

Insomnia

Tea made from aniseed is considered beneficial in the treatment of sleeplessness. It is prepared by boiling 375 ml of water and adding a teaspoon of aniseed. The water should be covered with a lid and allowed to simmer for 15 minutes. It should then be strained and taken hot or warm. Honey and hot milk will improve the taste. It should be sipped either after meals or before going to bed.

Precautions: Aniseed should not be boiled too long as it may lose its digestive properties and essential oil during the process.

Other Uses

Head Lice: Aniseed is used externally as an insecticide against small insects such as lice, mites and vermin. It also has fungicidal properties.

The seeds are used to flavour curries, sweets, cakes, cookies and biscuits. Anise oil is employed in medicine as an aromatic carminative to relieve flatulence. Being a mild expectorant, it is used as an ingredient of beverages and liqueurs. It is a popular flavouring agent for dental preparations and mouth washes.

Arjuna

Botanical Name: *Terminalia arjuna*
Indian Name: *Kahu*

Origin, Distribution and Composition

Arjuna is a dense tree attaining a height of 20 to 27 metres. It has long, cone-shaped round leaves and white bark which gives out a milky juice when cut. Mainly, the bark of the tree is used in medicines.

This tree has been named *Nadisarjja* in the early Sanskrit treatises, wherein its bark has been described as a cardiac tonic. Vagbhatta, an eminent physician of ancient India, was the first to prescribe bark of this tree for heart diseases. Later, Chakradatta, another great Indian physician, described it as a tonic and an astringent, and used it in heart diseases. He recommended its use either as a decoction with milk and treacle water (syrup) or as a *ghrita*, a preparation with *ghee* or clarified butter.

Arjuna tree is indigenous to India. It is found throughout the sub-Himalayan tracts, the Deccan regions, Myanmar and Sri Lanka. It grows chiefly along water channels or marshy belts.

The bark contains unusually large quantities of calcium, small amounts of aluminium and magnesium and tannins ---an astringent used in preparing leather and manufacturing ink. It also contains a crystalline compound arjunine, lactone, arjunetin, essential oil, sugars and colouring matter.

Healing Power and Curative Properties

The bark of the arjuna tree is a cardiac stimulant and has cooling and tonic effects. It is useful in arresting secretion or bleeding. It helps to relieve fever. It is also useful in removing calculi or stones formed in the urinary system; in promoting flow of bile; and in the healing of wounds.

Heart Disorders

The bark and preparations made from it are known to have a marked stimulant action on the heart. The practitioners of Indian system of medicine use them in conditions of cardiac failure and dropsy. Some practitioners of modern medicine believe in its stimulant effect on the heart and use it as a cardiac tonic. As a heart stimulant, either a decoction of the thick portion of the bark made with milk should be taken every morning on an empty stomach or its powder, in 0.75 to 2 grams doses, should be used with milk and jaggery.

Asthma

In *Ayurveda*, the bark of arjuna is considered beneficial in the treatment of asthma. According to this system, a fine powder of the bark is made and stored in a well-corked bottle. The patient suffering from asthma should keep fast on the day of the full moon. A dish of condensed milk and rice (*kheer*) should be prepared and placed where the moonlight falls upon it the whole night. During the early hours, 12 grams of the powdered bark should be sprinkled over the *kheer* and taken by the patient to his satisfaction. He should not sleep for at least 12 hours after consumption. This is believed to provide relief.

Fractures and Contusions

The bark of the tree helps the bones to regain their strength after a fracture. The powder of the bark can be given with honey.

Diarrhoea and Dysentery

A decoction of the bark taken in doses of 15 to 30 grams may relieve patients of diarrhoea or dysentery.

Acne

An ointment made by mixing the bark and honey applied over the affected area, can treat acne successfully.

Other Disorders

The juice of fresh leaves of the tree can be used beneficially in earache. Ashes of the bark is also prescribed in scorpion sting. The decoction of the herb is used as an astringent for cleaning sores, ulcers and syphilitic sores.

Other Uses

Aphrodisiac: The powder of the bark is an effective sex stimulant, if taken with milk regularly over a period of time.

Asafoetida

Botanical Name: *Ferula foetida, Ferula northex*
Indian Name: *Hing*

Origin, Distribution and Composition

Asafoetida is a resinous gum of a tall perennial herb, with robust carrot-shaped roots. It is dirty yellow in colour with a pungent smell. It is used as a flavouring agent and forms a constituent of many spice mixtures.

Asafoetida has several varieties which are distributed from the Mediterranean region to Central Asia. It is grown in Iran and Afghanistan. The other species, known botanically as Ferula northex, grow abundantly in Kashmir, Western Tibet and Afghanistan. It forms a good substitute for asafoetida.

An analysis of asafoetida shows it to consist of carbohydrates 67.8 per cent per 100 gms, moisture 16.0 per cent, protein 4.0 per cent, fat 1.1 per cent, minerals 7.0 per cent and fibre 4.1

per cent. Its mineral and vitamin contents include substantial calcium besides phosphorus, iron, carotene, riboflavin and niacin. Its calorific value is 297.

Asafoetida contains resin, gum, volatile oil and ash. The resin consists chiefly of asaresinotennol, free or combined with ferulic acid. Umbelliferone seems to be present in the combined state.

Healing Power and Curative Properties

Asafoetida has been held in great esteem amongst indigenous medicines from the earliest times in India. It is reputed as a drug which expels wind from the stomach and counteracts any spasmodic disorders. It is also a nervine stimulant, digestive agent and a sedative.

Respiratory Disorders

Asafoetida is useful in the treatment of respiratory disorders like whooping cough, asthma and bronchitis. About 3 to 6 centigrams of this gum, mixed with 2 teaspoons of honey, a quarter teaspoon of white onion juice and 1 teaspoon of betel leaf juice, taken thrice daily would keep the patient away from such disorders.

Hysteria

The herb is an effective remedy for hysteria. Inhaling this gum prevents hysterical attacks. An emulsion made by 2 grams of the gum with 120 ml of water is a valuable enema per rectum in treating hysteria, when oral dosage not advisable.

Impotency

The herb is beneficial in the treatment of impotency. About 6 centigrams of asafoetida should be fried in *ghee* and mixed with honey and a teaspoon of fresh latex of banyan tree. This mixture should be taken once daily for 40 days before sunrise. It is also considered a specific medicine for spermatorrhoea and premature ejaculation.

Children's Disorders

The herb is extensively used in the treatment of nervous disorders of children. There is an old European belief that a small piece of this gum, hung around a child's neck, would protect it from many diseases, especially germs which are sensitive to its particular odour.

Women's Ailments

The herb is considered useful in the treatment of several problems concerning women such as sterility, unwanted abortion, pre-mature labour, unusually painful, difficult and excessive menstruation and leucorrhoea. About 12 centigrams of gum fried in *ghee* mixed with 120 grams of goat's fresh milk and a tablespoon of honey, should be given thrice daily for a month. It excites the secretion of progestrone hormone.

Asafoetida is also useful for women after childbirth. Owing to its antiflatulent and digestive properties, the herb can be taken with beneficial results during the post-delivery period. In southern India, the powder of the herb mixed with rice is given to women after delivery.

Stomach Disorders

The herb is an effective remedy for several diseases of the stomach. It is one of the best remedies available for flatulence and is an essential ingredient for most of the digestive powders.

In case of flatulence and distension of the stomach, asafoetida should be dissolved in hot water and a pad of cloth steeped in it may be used for fomenting the abdomen.

Toothache

Asafoetida is useful in alleviating toothache. After being pestled in lemon juice, it is slightly heated. A cotton piece, soaked in the lotion and placed in the cavity of the tooth, relieves pain quickly.

Preparation and Doses: Asafoetida fried in *ghee* is administered either as a solution, emulsion or pills. The dose is 30 to 90 centigrams. The solution is made by thoroughly mixing 20 grams of the gum with half a litre of hot water. The dosage for adults is one to two tablespoons and one-fourth to half for children.

Other Uses

Antidote of Opium: The herb is used as an antidote of opium. Given in the same quantity as opium ingested by the patient, it will counteract the effect of the drug.

The gum resin is relished as a condiment in India and Iran where it is used to flavour curries, meatballs, dal and pickles. It is used in Europe and the United States in perfumes and for flavouring. The whole plant is used as a fresh vegetable.

Babul

Botanical Name: *Acacia arabica*
Indian Name: *Kikar*

Origin, Distribution and Composition

Acacia, popularly known as babul, is a large tree, upto 14 metres high, with thorns on its branches. It has darkish grey bark and yellow flowers in spherical heads.

Babul tree is indigenous to Sind in Pakistan. It occurs wild in India and tropical Africa. It is planted for its bark. The tree yields a gum, known as babul gum. The bark of babul tree contains tannin and gallic acid. The leaves and fruits of the tree also contain tannin and gallic acid.

Healing Power and Curative Properties

The leaves, the bark, the pods and the gum of the tree have medicinal virtues. The leaves and the bark are useful in arresting secretion or bleeding. The pods help remove catarrhal matter and phlegm from the bronchial tubes. The gum allays any irritation of the skin and soothes the inflamed membranes of the pharynx, alimentary canal and genito-urinary organs.

Diarrhoea

The various parts of babul tree are useful in diarrhoea of ordinary intensity. A mixture of equal parts of the tender leaves with white and black cumin seeds (*zeera*) can be administered in doses of 12 grams, thrice daily. An infusion made of the bark of the tree may also be taken thrice daily for the same purpose. The gum, used either in decoction or in syrup, is an effective medicine for diarrhoea.

Teeth Disorders

Chewing of fresh bark of this tree daily, helps strengthen loose teeth and arrest any bleeding from the gums. Dirty teeth can be cleaned effectively by brushing them with a' powder in which 60 grams of charcoal of babul wood, 24 grams of roasted alum and 12 grams of rock salt have been included.

Eczema

The bark of babul tree is useful in the treatment of eczema. About 25 grams each of this bark and the mango bark should be boiled in about 1 litre of water and the vapours allowed to foment the affected part. After the fomentation, the affected part should be anointed with *ghee*.

Tonsilitis

A decoction of the bark, mixed with rock salt, should be used as a gargle in treating tonsilitis.

Conjunctivitis

The leaves of babul tree are effective in the treatment of conjuctivitis. The leaves, ground to a paste, should be applied on the affected eyes at night, supported by a bandage which should be untied the next morning. This removes pain and redness.

Epiphora

The leaves are beneficial in treating epiphora— that is watering of the eyes, in which tears flow onto the cheeks due to abnormality of the tear drainage system. About 250 grams of leaves should be boiled in one and a quarter litre of water until only a quarter litre of water is left. This should then be filtered and kept in a well-corked bottle. The eye-lids should be painted morning and evening with this liquid.

Leucorrhoea

The bark of the tree is useful in leucorrhoea. Its decoction should be used as a vaginal douche for treating this disorder.

Other Uses

Sprematorrhoea: Fresh pods of babul tree are effective in sexual disorders like spermatorrhoea, frequent night discharges, loss of viscidity of the semen and premature ejaculation. In Ayurveda, a preparation made from the pods is considered highly beneficial in treating these disorders. It is prepared thus: about 1 to 1.5 metres of coarse cloth is spread evenly and its corners secured. The fresh pods of babul tree are pounded and their juice squeezed. This fresh juice is pasted on the cloth every morning and evening for at least 20 days until a 5-6 centimetres thick layer is formed on it. A small piece of this cloth weighing 5 to 9 grams is cut and boiled in a litre of cow's milk which is taken after adding brown sugar to taste.

It is also said to increase the power of retention of the semen. Even extremely debilitated patients suffering from the bad consequences of masturbation are believed to get rejuvenated by its use and attain normal retentive power. It improves the viscidity of the semen and is an excellent medicine for spermatorrhoea.

Another preparation made from the pods is also a very effective remedy for spermatorrhoea. Tender, seedless pods are dried in shade, powdered and mixed with an equal weight of brown sugar. Six grams of this mixture may be taken with milk in the morning.

Bael Fruit

Botanical Name: *Aegle marmelos*
Other English Names: *Stone apple, Bengal quince*
Indian Name: *Bel or Siriphal*

Origin, Distribution and Composition

The bael is a large tree, 8 to 10 metres in height. It has a big stout trunk, unusual branches with long, straight outgrowth, aromatic leaves, sweet scented and greenish-white flowers. The fruit is woody and smooth, 5 to 15 cm in diameter. It has numerous seeds which are densely covered with fibrous hair and are embedded in a thick aromatic pulp. The flesh is eaten fresh or dried.

Bael tree is held sacred by the Hindus. The history of this tree has been traced to Vedic period (2000 B.C. - 800 B.C.). The mention of bael fruit has been made in *Yajurveda*. The bael tree has great mythological significance and abounds in the vicinity of temples. The leaves of the tree are traditionally used as sacred offering to Lord Shiva, the God of health. Lord Shiva is believed to live under the bael tree. The bael tree is indigenous to India and is grown throughout the sub-continent as well as most countries of South-east Asia.

An analysis of the bael fruit shows that it consists of moisture 61.5 per cent, protein 1.8 per cent, fat 0.3 per cent, minerals 1.7 per cent, fibre 2.9 per cent and carbohydrates 31.8 per cent per 100 grams of edible portion. Its mineral and vitamin contents include calcium, phosphorus, iron, carotene, thiamin, riboflavin, niacin and vitamin C. Its calorific value is 137.

Several chemical constituents have been isolated and

identified from various parts of the bael tree. These include alkaloids, coumarins and steroids. The leaves contain skimianine, sterol and aegelin. The active constituent of the fruit is marmorosin, which is identical to imperatorin. Other coumarins contained in the fruits are altoimperatorin and B sitosterol. Roots of the tree have been found to contain psoralin, xanthotoxin, scopoletin and tembamide.

Healing Power and Curative Properties

The bael tree is one of the most useful medicinal plants of India. Its medicinal properties have been described in the ancient medical treatise in Sanskrit, *Charaka Samhita*. All parts of this tree—stem, bark, root, leaves and fruit at all stages of maturity —have medicinal virtues and have been used as medicine for a long time.

The fruit's medicinal value is very high when it just begins to ripen. The fruit is aromatic, cooling and laxative. It arrests secretion or bleeding. The unripe or half-ripe fruit is good for digestion. It is useful in preventing or curing scurvy. It also strengthens the stomach and promotes its action.

Constipation

Ripe bael fruit is regarded as best of all laxatives. It cleans and tones up the intestines. Its regular use for 2 or 3 months throws out even the old accumulated faecal matter. For best results, it should be taken in the form of *sherbet*, which is prepared from the pulp of the ripe fruit. After breaking the shell, the seeds are removed, with the contents spooned out and sieved. Milk and sugar are added to make it more palatable. The pulp of the ripe fruit can also be taken without the addition of milk or sugar. About 70 grams of the fruit will suffice for an adult.

Diarrhoea and Dysentery

The unripe or half-ripe fruit is perhaps the most effective remedy for chronic diarrhoea and dysentery where there is no fever. Best results are obtained by the use of dried bael or its powder. The bael fruit, when it is still green, is sliced and dried in the sun. The dried bael slices are powdered and preserved in airtight bottles. The unripe bael can also be baked and used with jaggery or brown sugar.

Peptic Ulcer

An infusion of bael leaves is regarded as an effective remedy for peptic ulcer. The leaves are soaked overnight in water. This water is strained and taken in the morning. The pain and discomfort are relieved when this treatment is continued for a few weeks. Bael leaves are rich in tannin which reduces inflammation and help in the healing of ulcers. Bael fruit taken in the form of a beverage also has great healing properties on account of its mucilage content. This forms a coating on the stomach mucosa and thus helps heal ulcers.

Ear Problems

The root of this tree is used as a home remedy for curing ear problems. A stiff piece of the root is dipped in *neem* oil and lighted. The oil that drips from the burning end is a highly effective medicine for ear problems. The antiseptic properties of *neem* combined with the astringent extract of bael root helps in curing infection, chronic inflammation and discharge.

Respiratory Disorders

A medicated oil prepared from bael leaves gives relief from recurrent colds and respiratory affections. The juice extracted from bael leaves is mixed with equal quantity of gingelly or sesame oil and heated thoroughly. A few seeds of black pepper and half a teaspoon of black cummin are added to the heated oil. It is then removed from the fire and stored for use when necessary. A teaspoon of this oil should be massaged into the scalp before a head bath. Its regular use builds up resistance to colds and coughs.

Precautions: The ripe fruit should not be taken regularly at a stretch. When used without a break, it produces atony of the intestines or lack of normal elasticity and consequent flatulence in the abdomen. The bael fruit should also not be taken in excess at a time, as excessive intake may produce a sensation of heaviness in the stomach.

The *sherbet* made of bael must not be very thin. It should be viscous so that it can be thoroughly chewed. It may produce heaviness in the stomach, if taken hurriedly.

Bamboo

Botanical Name: *Bambusa bambos*
Indian Name: *Bans*

Origin, Distribution and Composition

The bamboo is a perennial tree which grows upto a height of 12 metres with its trunk 8 to 15 cm in diameter. Every year, between July and October, new shoots sprout at the base of the tree. Bamboo trees are always found in clusters.

The stem of the tree is round, smooth and hollow. Nodes are swollen. The tree has no branches but, the lower portions, that is, three-fourths of the tree, have more spines between each node. It has simple, shiny, thin, stiff, smooth and dark green leaves. Flowers are found in bunch and seeds resemble the corn of wheat, in shape.

Bamboo is presumed to have originated in Asia. The tree grows wild throughout most parts of India, especially in the hilly forests of western and southern India but is cultivated only in the lower Himalayas and in the valleys of the Ganges and Indus.

An analysis of bamboo shows that it contains moisture 88.8 per cent, protein 3.9 per cent, fat 0.5 per cent, minerals 1.1 per cent and carbohydrates 5.7 per cent per 100 grams of its edible portion. Calcium, phosphorus, iron, thiamine, riboflavin, niacine and vitamin C are amongst its vitamin and minerals. Its calorific value is 43.

Bamboo leaves are a rich source of hydrocyanic and benzoic acids. Tender bamboo-shoots contain various enzymes such as nuclease, deamidase, proteolytic enzyme, amylase, amigdalin splitting and silicon splitting enzymes. Besides, the juice of the pressed bamboo-shoots possesses protease activity which helps digestion of proteins.

Healing Power and Curative Properties

The leaves of bamboo tree are stimulant, aromatic and tonic. They are useful in counteracting spasmodic disorders, and arrest secretion or bleeding. They are also an effective aphrodisiac. The leaves do not have any prominent taste.

Stomach Disorders

The leaves are beneficial in the treatment of stomach troubles. They are useful in strengthening the stomach and

35

promoting its action. The young shoots of the tree are also useful in stomach disorders. Pickled or cooked, they serve as an appetizer. In many parts of India, the leaves of the tree are used in the form of decoction to treat diarrhoea.

Respiratory Disorders

The tender shoots are useful in the treatment of respiratory diseases. Decoction of the shoots should be taken with a tablespoon of honey once or twice daily.

Menstrual Disorders

A decoction of the leaves as an emmanagouge would stimulate menstruation. It promotes and regulates the menstrual periods. A decoction of the nodes of the bamboo stem is also useful for this purpose.

Intestinal Worms

The leaves are useful in killing intestinal worms, especially threadworms. They should be taken in the form of decoction.

Wounds and Ulcers

A poultice of the tender shoots is used for cleaning wounds and maggot-infested sores. Decoction or juice of the fresh bamboo leaves is applied as a medicine in such ulcers.

Dosage: The juice of 35 grams of fresh leaves may be taken twice daily either alone or mixed with any other juice. The decoction extracted from 70 grams of leaves may be used by itself. About 120 ml of the juice extracted from very tender shoots may be taken twice daily.

Other Uses

Abortion, Pregnancy and Post-Delivery Use: Decoction of the tender bamboo-shoots, mixed with palm jaggery (*tad-ka-gud*), is given once or twice a day for a week to cause abortion during the first month of pregnancy. The same preparation can be used in the last month of pregnancy to induce labour. Its use after the childbirth eases the process of the expulsion of the placenta and prevents excessive loss of blood. It is a safe substitute for ergot in such conditions.

Bamboo shoots are used as food in various ways. They are used in preparation such as bamboo candy, bamboo chutney and canning of bamboo in syrups.

Banyan

Botanical Name: *Ficus bengalensis*
Indian Name: *Bar*

Origin, Distribution and Composition

The banyan tree is well known all over India. The tree has what is known as the 'aerial roots'; its branches drop to the ground, take roots again, and send out more twisting and trailing branches, thus extending the growth of the tree indefinitely. It has smooth, shining, rather stiff and leathery leaves, broadly oval in shape. The flowers and fruits are inconspicious, very minute, many of them being held together in the fig, which is a sort of pouch that contains hundreds of flowers or fruits.

The name Banyan tree in English seems to have been given by Europeans in the Persian Gulf to a particular tree of this species under which Banias or members of the Indian merchant class used to congregate for worship and business. Gradually, the name spread to indicate all the species of this tree. From time immemorial, poets and mystics of India have been eloquent in singing the praises of this tree. It is now one of the commonest trees planted along the country roads, shrines, or uncultivated fields in India.

The leaves of the banyan tree yield ficusin and bergaptene. The latex of the tree is very toxic.

Healing Power and Curative Properties

The banyan has many medicinal properties. It is used in traditional medicine for the treatment of several ailments. The bark and leaf buds of the tree are useful in arresting secretion or bleeding. The fruit exercises a soothing effect on the skin and mucous membranes, alleviates swelling and pain, and serve as a mild purgative. It is also nutritious.

Diarrhoea and Dysentery

The leaf buds of the banyan tree are beneficial in the treatment of chronic diarrhoea and dysentery. The buds should be soaked in water overnight and taken as infusion in the treatment of these diseases. The latex is also useful in the treatment of diarrhoea and dysentery.

Piles

A few drops of the latex of the banyan tree mixed in milk and taken daily helps to cure bleeding piles. With this treatment, the diet of the patient should contain liberal quantities of green vegetables especially fenugreek and *manattakkali* or black nightshade leaves.

Female Sterility

Tender roots of the banyan tree are considered beneficial in the treatment of female sterility. These roots should be dried in the shade and finely powdered. This powder should be mixed 5 times its weight, with milk, and taken at night for 3 consecutive nights after menstruation cycle every month till the conception takes place. No other food should be taken with this.

Leucorrhoea

A regular douching of the genital tract with a decoction of the bark of the banyan tree and the fig tree is helpful in leucorrhoea. A tablespoon each of the powders of the bark of the two trees should be boiled in a litre of water till it is reduced to about half. Douching with the lukewarm decoction will keep the tissues of vaginal tract healthy.

Teeth Disorders

Cleaning the teeth with the aerial roots of the banyan is beneficial in preventing teeth and gum disorders. As one chews the stick and brushes, the astringent secretion from the root-stick cleanses and strengthens the teeth and gums.

Rheumatism

The latex is commonly used locally for rheumatism, pain and lumbago.

Skin Disorders

A hot poultice of the leaves can be applied with beneficial results to abscesses to promote suppuration and to hasten their breaking. The milky juice from the fresh green leaves is useful in destroying warts. The latex is commonly used locally for sores, ulcers and bruises.

Kibes

Those who do not wear socks and shoes suffer from cracking of heels, a condition known as kibes. The best way to deal with this condition is to fill the cracks with the sap of the banyan tree.

Other Diseases

An infusion of the bark is a specific medicine for diabetes. The tender ends of the aerial roots can be taken in obstinate vomiting.

Belleric Myroblan

Botanical Name: *Terminalia belerica*
Indian Name: *Bahera*

Origin, Distribution and Composition

Belleric myroblan is a large tree, often with buttresses. It has large leaves, 10 to 25 cm long, clustered near ends of branches; small pale green foul-smelling flowers in simple spikes and egg-shaped, brownish long fruits densely covered with hair.

The word Belleric is taken from the scientific name which distinguishes this myroblan from the other one, that is, chebulic myroblan, *(harad)*. The dried fruits of the tree constitute the drug *bahera*. The trade name *bahera* is based on the Indian name of the tree.

This tree is indigenous to India. It occurs almost throughout the country up to about 1,000 metres excepting the dry regions of Western India. It is more common in mixed deciduous forests.

The herb contains substantial amounts of tannin substances.

Healing Power and Curative Properties

The herb is bitter in taste. It is a tonic and a laxative and arrests secretion or bleeding. It is also useful in reducing fevers. The *bahera* fruit is one of the three constituents of the famous Indian preparation *triphala*, the other two being embelica myroblan *(amla)* and chebulic myroblan *(harad)*.

Coughs

Belleric myroblan is a household remedy for coughs. A mixture of the pulp of the fruit, salt, long pepper and honey is administered in the treatment of cough. The fried fruit covered with wheat flour and roasted, is another popular remedy for cough and catarrh.

Stomach Disorders

The herb is extremely useful in stomach disorders such as indigestion and diarrhoea. A decoction or infusion of 1 to 3 grams of the pulp of the fruit should be administered in these disorders.

Sore Throat

The same mixture as for cough treatment is also a useful remedy for sore throat and hoarseness of voice. The fried fruit is another remedy for treating sore throat. It should be given in the same manner as for cough.

Chronic Constipation

The half ripe fruit is considered useful as a purgative. It can be used beneficially in the treatment of chronic constipation. However, the ripe and dried fruit has the opposite property.

Intestinal Worms

Belleric myroblan, mixed with the seeds of butea *(palash)* is very effective anthelmintic. It should be taken in doses of one teaspoon thrice a day. It helps remove all intestinal parasites.

Eye Disorders

The herb can be applied on the eyes as a soothing lotion. Its fine powder can be used beneficially in epiphora—that is watering of the eyes, in which tears flow onto the cheeks due to abnormality of the tear drainage system.

Other Diseases

Belleric myroblan can be used with gratifying result as a brain tonic. It is also useful in leprosy, piles, dropsy and fever.

Betel Leaves

Botanical Name: *Piper betle*
Indian Name: *Pan*

Orgin, Distribution and Composition

The betel plant is a slender, aromatic creeper, rooting at the nodes. The branches of the plant are swollen at the nodes. The plant has alternate, heart-shaped, smooth, shining and long-stalked leaves, with pointed apex. It has five to seven ribs arising from the base; minute flowers and one-seeded spherical small berries.

The use of betel leaf can be traced as far back as two thousand years. It is described in the most ancient historic book of Sri Lanka, *Mahavasma*, written in Pali.

Betel is a native of central and eastern Malaysia. It spread at a very early date throughout tropical Asia and later to Madagascar and East Africa. In India, it is widely cultivated in Tamil Nadu, Madhya Pradesh, West Bengal, Orissa, Maharashtra and Uttar Pradesh. Offering betel morsel *(pan-supari)* to guests in Indian subcontinent is a common courtesy.

An analysis of the betel leaf shows it to consist of moisture 85.4 per cent, protein 3.1 per cent, fat 0.8 per cent, minerals 2.3 per cent, fibre 2.3 per cent and carbohydrates 6.1 per cent per 100 grams. Its minerals and vitamin contents are calcium, carotene, thiamine, riboflavin, niacin and vitamin C. Its calorific value is 44.

Recent studies have shown that betel leaves contain tannins, sugar and diastases and an essential oil. The essential oil is a light yellow liquid of aromatic odour and sharp burning in taste. It contains a phenol called chavicol which has powerful antiseptic properties. The alkaloid arakene in it, has properties resembling cocaine in some respects.

Healing Power and Curative Properties

Betel leaf has been used from ancient times as an aromatic stimulant and antiflatulent. It is useful in arresting secretion or bleeding and is an aphrodisiac. Its leaf is used in several common household remedies.

Scanty or Obstructed Urination

Betel leaf juice is credited with diuretic properties. Its juice, mixed with dilute milk and sweetened slightly, helps in easing urination.

Weakness of Nerves

Betel leaves are beneficial in the treatment of nervous pains, nervous exhaustion and debility. The juice of a few betel leaves, with a teaspoon of honey, will serve as a good tonic. A teaspoon of this can be taken twice a day.

Headaches

The betel leaf has analgesic and cooling properties. It can be applied with beneficial results over the painful area to relieve intense headache.

Respiratory Disorders

Betel leaves are useful in pulmonary affection in childhood and old age. The leaves, soaked in mustard oil and warmed, may be applied to the chest to relieve cough and difficulty in breathing.

Constipation

In the case of constipation in children, a suppository made of the stalk of betel leaf dipped in castor oil can be introduced in the rectum. This instantly relieves constipation.

Sore Throat

Local application of the leaves is effective in treating sore throat. The crushed fruit or berry should be mixed with honey and taken to relieve irritating cough[1].

Inflammation

Applied locally, betel leaves are beneficial in the treatment of inflammation such as arthritis and orchitis, that is inflammation of the testes.

Wounds

Betel leaves can be used to heal wounds. The juice of a few leaves should be extracted and applied on the wound. Then a betel leaf should be wrapped over and bandaged. The wound will heal up with a single application within 2 days.

Boils

The herb is also an effective remedy for boils. A leaf is gently warmed till it gets softened, and is then coated with a layer of castor oil. The oiled leaf is spread over the inflamed part. This leaf has to be replaced, every few hours. After a few applications, the boil will rupture draining all the purulent matter. The application can be made at night and removed in the morning.

---

1. R.N. Chopra, *et al*, *Indigenous drugs of India*, p. 371 Acedemic Publishers, Calcutta.

Lumbago

A hot poultice of the leaves or their juice mixed with some bland oil such as refined coconut oil can be applied to the loins with beneficial results in lumbago.

Problem of Breast Milk Secretion

The application of leaves smeared with oil is said to promote secretion of milk when applied on the breasts during lactation.

Precautions: Cancer of the mouth and lips has been found to be more frequent in areas where the betel chewing habit is widely prevalent. Other ill-effects of *pan*-chewing like dyspepsia, pyorrhoea, cancer of the tongue and cheeks have also been observed amongst excessive chewers.

Other Uses

Aphrodisiac: *Pan-supari*, especially the *pan*, is prescribed by Ayurvedic physicians as an aphrodisiac. Partly owing to its deodorant, aphrodisiac, and invigorating properties, *pan-supari* came to form a part of the ritual with which a wife welcomed her husband.

The betel leaves are chewed together with betel nut as a masticatory. In its simplest form, sliced betel nut is wrapped in a betel leaf, smeared with lime and chewed. Often though, a clove and other spices such as cinnamon and cardamom are added. When chewed after meals, it sweetens the breath and acts as a gentle stimulant.

Bishop's Weed

Botanical Name: *Trachyspermum ammi*
Indian Name: *Ajwain or Omum*

Origin, Distribution and Composition

Bishop's weed is a small, erect, annual shrub, with soft fine hairs. It has many branched leafy stems; feather-like leaves 2.5 cm long; and 4 to 12 ray flowerheads, each bearing 6 to 16 flowers. The fruits are minute, egg-shaped and greyish.

The trade name *ajwain* is based on the Indian name which is derived from *adarjawan*. *Ajwain* or Bishop's weed has been used as a carminative medicine from the time of Charaka and

43

Sushruta. Even Greek physicians like Dioscrides and Gelen used it in various carminative medicines. Some very valuable Unani medicines are prepared from *ajwain* seeds.

Bishop's weed is cultivated in Iran, Egypt, Afghanistan and India.

An analysis of the *ajwain* seeds shows them to consist of moisture 7.4 per cent, protein 17.1 per cent, fat 21.8 per cent, minerals 7.9 per cent, fibre 21.2 per cent and carbohydrates 24.6 per cent per 100 grams. Calcium, phosphorus, iron, carotene, thiamine, riboflavin and niacin are amongst the vitamins and minerals in it. Its calorific value is 363.

Steam distillation of crushed seeds yields an essential oil which is valued considerably in medicine on account of the presence of thymol. The oil was, for a long time, the chief source of thymol.

Healing Power and Curative Properties

The seeds are stimulant and are useful in counteracting spasmodic disorders. The oil of *ajwain* is an almost colourless to brownish liquid with characteristic odour and a sharp hot taste. If the liquid is allowed to remain undisturbed, a part of the thymol may separate from the crystals, which is sold in Indian markets under the name of *ajwain ka phul* or *sat ajwain*. It is much valued in medicine as it has nearly all the properties ascribed to the *ajwain* seeds.

Gastro-Intestinal Disorders

Bishop's weed has long been used in indigenous medicine for the treatment of diarrhoea, dysentery, atonic dyspepsia, cholera, colic, flatulence and indigestion. For relieving flatulence, dyspepsia and spasmodic disorders, the seeds may be eaten with betel leaves. A teaspoon of these seeds with a little rock-salt is a household remedy for indigestion.

The volatile oil extracted from the seeds is also useful in cholera, flatulent colic, diarrhoea, atonic dyspepsia and indigestion. It is usually given in doses of 1 to 3 drops. *Omum* water, that is, the water distilled from the seeds, is an excellent carminative that relieves flatulence and is antispasmodic in colic and flatulent dyspepsia. It is also administered in the early stages of cholera in doses of 30 to 60 grams to check vomiting.

In case of colic, *ajwain*, dry ginger and black salt in the

44

proportion of 1 : 1/2 : 1/4 should be ground together and taken in three gram doses with warm water. In case of flatulence, *ajwain* and dried ginger in equal weight may be soaked in two-and-half times the quantity of lime juice. This is then dried and powdered with a little black salt. About two grams of this powder is taken with warm water.

Respiratory Disorders

A mixture of the seeds and buttermilk is an effective remedy for relieving difficult expectoration caused by dried up phlegm. The seeds are also efficacious in bronchitis. A hot fomentation with the seeds is a popular household remedy for asthma. Chewing a pinch of *ajwain* seeds with a crystal of common salt and a clove is a very effective remedy for cough caused by acute pharyngitis in influenza.

Common Cold

Bishop's weed is an effective common cold remedy. It has a remarkable power to open up clogged and congested nasal passages. A tablespoon of seeds crushed and tied up in a cloth bundle can be used for inhalation. A similar bundle placed near the pillow, while sleeping, also relieves nasal congestion. For infants and small children, a small pouch can be pinned to their dress under the chin when they are sleeping. In case of adults, a teaspoon of the seeds can be put in boiling water and the vapours inhaled.

Migraine

The seeds are useful in the treatment of migraine and delerium. They should either be smoked or sniffed frequently to obtain relief.

Rheumatism

The oil extracted from the seeds is beneficial in the treatment of rheumatic and neuralgic pains. It should be applied on the affected parts.

Mouth Disorders

An infusion of the seeds mixed with common salt is an effective gargle in acute pharyngitis, sore and congested throat and hoarseness of the voice due to colds or shouting.

Earache

The herb is beneficial in earache. About half a teaspoon of

the seeds is heated in 30 ml of milk till the essence of the seeds permeate the milk. The milk is then filtered and used as ear drops. It decreases congestion and relieves pain.

In case of pain caused by boils in the ear, 3 grams each of *ajwain* seeds and garlic are boiled together in 40 grams of sesame oil till they turn red. The oil is then strained and cooled to body temperature, and used as ear drops.

Other Uses

Aphrodisiac: *Ajwain* seeds, combined with the kernel of tamarind seeds are an effective aphrodisiac. These should be fried in equal quantity of pure ghee, powdered and preserved in airtight containers. A teaspoon of this powder, mixed with a tablespoon of honey, taken daily with milk before retiring, makes an excellent aphrodisiac. It increases virility and cures premature ejaculation.

The greyish brown fruits or seeds are used as a spice, in flavouring numerous foods, as anti-oxidants, preservatives and in medicine.

Black Nightshade

Botanical Name: *Solanum nigrum*
Indian Name: *Makoy or Manathakkali*

Origin, Distribution and Composition

The black nightshade, also known as sunberry or wonder cherry, is a small, erect and delicate annual herb. It forms a spreading crown, grows diffusedly with several arching branches upto one metre in height. The stems and branches are smooth and soft. The plant has alternate, egg-shaped, elliptic leaves; white, cream or violet flowers in clusters, purple or black fruit when ripe; with blue or black seeds.

The black nightshade is a native of West Africa, but is now grown all over India as well.

An analysis of black nightshade or *manathakkali leaves* shows them to consist of moisture 82.1 per cent, protein 5.9 per cent, fat 1.0 per cent, minerals 2.1 per cent and carbohydrates 8.9 per cent per 100 grams. The minerals and vitamins presents in it include calcium, phosphorus, iron, riboflavin, niacin and vitamin C. Its calorific value is 68.

The plant and the fruit contain toxic alkaloid solanine and saponin. Feeding experiments on sheep for toxicity, however, showed negative results.

Healing Power and Curative Properties

The black nightshade is used as an important ingredient in several Indian medicines. It is a valuable cardiac tonic. It corrects disordered processes of nutrition by which the organism ingests, digests, absorbs, transports, utilises and excretes food substances, and restores the normal function of the system. It also reduces excitement, irritation and pain.

The leaves of the plant are mildly bitter, which becomes less pronounced after cooking. The fruits of the plant are of tonic value and serve as an effective laxative. They improve appetite.

Dropsy

The plant is beneficial in the treatment of dropsy. It increases the secretion and discharge of urine. Either it can be used as decoction or as a vegetable in the treatment of this disease. An extract of the leaves and stem, in doses of 6 to 8 ml., can also be taken.

Fevers

Manathakkali leaves are useful in fevers. A syrup of the vegetable can be given as a cooling drink. To induce copious perspiration, a hot infusion of 0.75 to 1.25 decigrams, of dried leaves can be used. The fruits of the plant can also be given with beneficial results in fevers.

Stomach Disorders

The leaves are effective in the treatment of digestive disorders. The raw juice of the leaves can be used alone or mixed with other juices or liquids. It is used in stomach disorders like flatulence, peptic ulcers and colitis. An infusion of the plant is useful in dysentery and other stomach ailments.

Asthma

The plant helps in removing catarrhal matter and phlegm from the bronchial tubes in asthma patients. The fruits of the plant can also be used beneficially in treating asthma.

Skin Disorders

The plant is useful in chronic skin diseases. The juice extracted from the plant should be given in doses of 180 to 210 ml.

The juice can also be applied locally on the affected parts in chronic skin disease such as acne, eczema and psoriasis. As an anodyne or pain reliever, a decoction of the plant can be used for washing inflamed, irritated and painful parts of the body.

A paste of the plant serves as a useful applicant over corrosive ulcers, pustules and suppurating syphilitic ulcers, severe burns, herpes and rheumatic joints. Green fruits of the plant can be ground and applied locally on ringworms with gratifying results. A juice or poultice of leaves can be effectively applied on eruptive skin diseases, whitlow and burns.

Other Diseases

Hot leaves can be applied with gratifying results over swollen and painful scrotum and testicles. A juice or poultice of the leaves is an efficacious application over rheumatic and gouty joints, corrosive ulcers and tumours. A decoction of the leaves can be used to wash tumours and inflamed, irritated and painful parts or the body.

Other Uses

Manathakkali leaves are popularly used as a vegetable. The leaves blend well with other greens and pulses. The juice of the leaves can be mixed with medium like coconut water, coconut milk, butter-milk, cow's milk and fruit juice.

Butea

Botanical Name: *Butea monosperma*
Indian Name: *Palas*

Origin, Distribution and Composition

Butea, also known as "flame of the forest", is a well known tree of India. The scarlet and orange flowers of the tree make its name appropriate. Butea is a medium-sized tree, with compound leaves. The leaves fall in winter and flowers bloom in February-March in small but dense clusters generally on leafless branches, and the tree appears to be aflame. The fruits are flat pods, with a single seed in each fruit.

This herb is indigenous to India. The trade name butea, is based on the scientific name of the plant. The tree is found chiefly in the mixed or dry deciduous forests of Central and Western India.

The red-coloured gum, called Bengal kino or butea gum, obtained from the tree, is rich in gallic and tannic acids. The seeds contain a yellow fixed oil called moodooga oil or kino-tree oil, small quantities of a resin and large quantities of a water-soluble albuminoid. Fresh seeds contain proteolytic and lipolytic enzymes. The flowers contain glucosides, butrin, butin and neteroside. A number of fatty acids have been isolated from the oil.

Healing Power and Curative Properties

The butea gum, the seeds and leaves of the tree have medicinal properties. The leaves of the tree are tonic and aphrodisiac. They are useful in arresting secretion or bleeding.

Diarrhoea and Dysentery

The gum of the tree is useful in the treatment of diarrhoea and dysentry. Its action is however mild, particularly suitable for children and women of delicate disposition. It is given in doses of 3 decigrams to 2 grams, with a few decigrams of aromatics. The leaves can be chewed orally during the ailment. Infusion or decoction of the gum as a rectal enema would yield instant relief. Fresh juice of the leaves is also useful in these diseases.

Intestinal Worms

The seeds are administered internally, either in the form of powder or made into a paste with honey as an anthelmintic to kill intestinal worms. They are specially useful in the treatment of roundworms and tapeworms. Recent experiments have confirmed their effectiveness in eliminating round worms. About a gram of the seeds mixed with honey can be given thrice a day for 3 days to treat intestinal worms. On the fourth day, a dose of castor oil may be administered to evacuate the bowels.

Skin Disorders

The seeds are beneficial in the treatment of certain skin

diseases. The seeds, ground and mixed with lemon juice, can be daubed on dhobi's itch—an eczema-type of skin disorder, characterized by itching. They can also be applied with gratifying results on ringworms. A hot poultice of the leaves can be applied to resolve boils, pimples, tumorous piles, ulcers and swellings. The crushed seeds can be used for killing maggots in wounds and sores.

Diabetes

The leaves of the tree are very useful in diabetes. They reduce blood sugar and are useful in glycosuria--that is, the presence of a large amount of glucose in urine.

Leucorrhoea

The leaves are also beneficial in the treatment of leucorrhoea. Decoction or infusion of leaves should be used as a vaginal douche for this purpose.

Sore Throat

The leaves are useful in congested and septic throat. A decoction of the leaves obtained by boiling them in water, should be used as a mouth-wash in the treatment of this disorder.

Retention of Urine

The leaves are useful in treating the difficulty of retention of urine. The pubic region should be fomented with the leaves in this disorder.

Caraway Seeds

Botanical Name: *Carum carvi*
Indian Name: *Siya jeera*

Origin, Distribution and Composition

The caraway plant is a biennial herb usually with a fleshy root and slender, branched stems. It has feather-like leaves divided into very narrow segments and small white flowers. The fruit, when ripe, splits into narrow, elongated carpels, which are curved, pointed at the ends and have four longitudinal ridges on the surface. The dried fruits or seeds, brown in colour, are hard and sharp to touch. They have a pleasant odour, aromatic flavour, somewhat sharp taste and leave a somewhat warm feeling in the mouth.

Caraway's qualities were recognised by the ancient Egyptians, Greeks and Romans. The herb was widely used in the Middle Ages. It has been used for centuries in breads and cakes, and with baked fruit, especially roasted apples. Because caraway was said to prevent lovers from straying, it was once an essential ingredient in love potions. The seeds of caraway were prescribed for bringing bloom to the cheeks of pale-faced young maidens.

The caraway seed is native to north and central Europe and West Asia. In India, it grows wild in the north Himalayan region. The herb is cultivated as a winter crop on the plains and summer one in Kashmir, Kumaon, Garhwal and Chamba at altitudes of 2,740 to 3,660 metres.

An analysis of caraway seeds shows it to contain appreciable moisture, protein, fat, substantial amount of carbohydrates besides ash, calcium, phosphorus, sodium, potassium, iron, thiamine, riboflavin and niacin. It also contains vitamins C and A. Its calorific value is 465 per 100 gram.

A valuable essential oil, containing substantial amounts of carvone, is obtained from caraway seeds. This oil is colourless or pale yellow with a strong odour and flavour of the fruit. The volatile oil contains a mixture of ketone, carvone, a terpene and traces of carvacrol.

Healing Power and Curative Properties

The caraway seeds, leaves and roots are considered useful in activating the glands, besides increasing the action of the kidneys. It is characterised as an excellent 'house cleaner' for the body. Caraway oil is used in medicine to relieve flatulence. It is also used to correct the nauseating and griping effects of some medicines.

Stomach Disorders

Caraway seeds are useful in strengthening the functions of stomach. They relieve flatulence and are useful in flatulent colic, countering any possible adverse effects of medicines. However, the volatile oil of the seeds is employed more often than the seeds. For flatulence, a cup of tea made from caraway seeds taken thrice a day, after meals, will give relief. This tea is prepared by adding a teaspoon of caraway seeds in 1.5 to 2 litres

51

of boiling water and allowing it to simmer on a slow fire for 15 minutes. It is then strained and sipped hot or warm.

Hookworms

Carvone, isolated from caraway oil, is used as anthelmintic, especially in removing hookworms from the intestines.

Scabies

A dilute solution, containing small amounts of the oil of the caraway and alcohol mixed in 75 parts of castor oil is considered beneficial in the treatment of scabies. The solution should be taken orally.

Bad Breath

Caraway seed oil is used orally in overcoming bad breath or insipid taste.

Other Uses

Caraway is widely used for flavouring breads, biscuits, cakes and cheese. It is also used as an ingredient in sausages and as a seasoning and pickling spices. Caraway oil is useful chiefly for flavouring purposes and in medicine as a carminative to relieve flatulence.

Cardamom

Botanical Name: *Elettaria Cardamomum*
Indian Name: *Chhoti elaichi*

Origin, Distribution and Composition

Cardamom is the "queen of spices", second only to black pepper, the "king of spices". It is one of the most valued spices in the world.

Cardamom grows as a perennial herb with thick, fleshy rhizomes or underground stems shooting leafy roots and with leafy stems. It has very large leaves, white or pale green three-celled flowers, many-seeded pale green to yellow fruits and triangular brownish-black seeds.

The dried cardamom fruits of the plant constitute the drug. They have a pleasant aroma with a characteristic, slightly pungent taste. They leave a warm feeling in the mouth. It is the seeds, taken out from the fruits, which produce the warm sensation.

Cardamoms are mentioned by Theophrastus in the fourth century BC and five centuries later by Dioscoredes. By 1000 AD, they were an article of trade from India westwards.

Cardamom is indigenous to South India. It grows wild in the rich moist forests of Mysore, Coorg, Wynaad, Travancore and Cochin. Cultivation is still limited to a few countries, mainly India, Sri Lanka and Guatemala.

An analysis of the cardamom capsule shows it to consist of carbohydrates, moisture, protein, ether extract, volatile oil, crude fibre, calcium, phosphorus and iron.

The seeds contain a volatile oil. The principal constituents of the volatile oil are cineol, terpineol, terpinene, limonene, sabinene, and terpineol in the form of formic and acetic acids.

Healing Power and Curative Properties

The aroma and therapeutic properties of cardamom are due to its volatile oil. Tinctures of cardamom are used chiefly in medicines to relieve flatulence and for strengthening digestion activities.

Digestive Disorders

Cardamom reduces the air and water elements, increases appetite and soothes the mucous membrane. It relieves gas and heart-burn caused by garlic and onion. Ground cardamom seed mixed with ginger, cloves and coriander, is an effective remedy for indigestion. A tea made from cardamom is valuable in headache caused by indigestion.

Bad Breath

The aromatic flavour in cardamom is a breath freshener. A few seeds chewed for a brief period will remove foul smell.

Genito-Urinary Disorders

Its powdered seeds mixed with a tablespoon of banana leaf and *amla* juice taken thrice a day, will serve as an excellent diuretic for the treatment of gonorrhoea, cystitis, nephritis, burning micturation or urination and scanty urination.

Depression

Powdered seeds of cardamon are boiled in water with tea. It gives a very pleasing aroma to the tea. This can be used as a remedy in the treatment of depression.

Impotency

The herb is useful in sexual dysfunctions like impotency and premature ejaculation. A pinch of powdered cardamom seeds boiled in milk and sweetened with honey every night would yield excellent results. Excessive use of cardamom at times may lead to impotency.

Oral Disorders

Gargling with an infusion of cardamom and cinnamon cures pharyngitis, sore-throat, relaxes uvula, or the fleshy conical portion at the back of the tongue, and hoarseness during the infective stage of influenza. Its daily gargle protects one from the flu.

Other Uses

Hiccups: An infusion made by boiling a couple of pounded whole cardamoms in a cup of water along with 5 leaves of mint is useful in relieving hiccups.

In India, cardamom is used as masticatory and often included in *pan-supari*. It is used for flavouring curries, cakes, bread and for other culinary purposes, like flavouring coffee or confectionery.

The essential oil of cardamom is used for pharmaceutical purposes, perfumery, flavouring liquers and bitters, in the preparation of tincture and as a stimulant.

Cassia

Botanical Name: *Cassia fistula*
Indian Name: *Amaltas*

Origin, Distribution and Composition

Cassia or purging cassia is one of the most beautiful trees of India. It is a small to medium-sized tree with compound leaves and large, shining, dark green leaflets. It has bright yellow flowers in very large, hanging branches and black or shining dark brown, 50 to 60 cm long almost cylindrical fruits.

The tree is also known as Indian Laburnum owing to its resemblance in colour and profusion of flowers with the European Laburnum. The trade name is based on its scientific name but the specific name fistula, which means a shepherd's pipe, refers to the shape of its fruit.

The cassia tree is indigenous to India. It is very decorative and is found throughout India upto an altitude of about 1500 metres. It is more common in moist or evergreen forests.

The leaves of the tree contain anthraquinone derivatives and very little tannin. The root bark, besides tannin, contains phlobaphenes and oxy-anthraquinone substance; the pulp contains rhein, the major anthraquinone derivative, a small amount of volatile oil, three waxy substances and a resinous substance.

Healing Power and Curative Properties

Nearly all parts of the tree have medicinal properties. The fruits are, however, most important and are included in the Indian Pharmaceutical Codex.

Constipation

The pulp from the fruits, called cassia pulp, is a well-known laxative, and is used in the treatment of constipation. It can be safely taken even by children and expectant mothers. About 50 grams of the pulp is soaked in water overnight. It is then strained in the morning and taken with 25 grams of sugar.

The pulp of cassia is a mild, pleasant and safe purgative. Approximately four grams of the pulp is taken with an equal quantity of sugar or tamarind. As a purgative, 30 to 60 grams are required, but this quantity may cause colic, nausea and flatulence. It is therefore generally used in combination with other drugs, preferably in mixture with the leaves of senna, botanically known as *cassia angustifolia*.

Common Cold

The root of the tree is useful in common cold. In case of running nose, smoke from the burning root can be inhaled. It encourages a copious nasal discharge and provides relief.

Fevers

The root of the tree is a tonic and useful in reducing fever. An alcoholic extract of the root-bark is used for black water fever.

Intestinal Disorders

For children suffering from flatulence, the cassia pulp can

be applied around the navel to ensure evacuation. Mixed with linseed or almond oil, it can be massaged on the stomach for easing the bowel movements.

Aguesia

The pulp of cassia is very useful in ageusia or loss of sense of taste due to excessive use of opium or cocaine. About 24 grams of the pulp is mixed with a quarter litre of hot milk and used as a mouthwash to treat this syndrome.

Skin Disorders

The leaves of the tree are useful in relieving irritation of the skin and in alleviating swellings and pains. Their juice or paste serves as a useful dressing for ringworm and inflammation of the hands or feet caused by exposure to cold. They also relieve dropsical swellings due to excessive accumalation of fluid in the body tissue. Its leaves can be rubbed beneficially on affected parts for relief from rheumatism and facial paralysis.

Other Uses

Its flowers are at times consumed as vegetables by certain hill tribes in India.

Castor Seeds

Botanical Name: *Ricinus communis*
Indian Name: *Arandi*

Origin, Distribution and Composition

The castor is a small annual plant. It ranges from 1 to 7 metres in height. It has well-developed roots, with green and reddish stems which become hollow with age. The fruit is a spherical capsule with small grey seeds with brown spots.

Castor seeds were an important item of commerce in ancient Egypt. It has been found in tombs dating from 4000 BC. In India too, castor has been used since ancient times. In the *Susruta Atharvaveda*, dating back to 2000 BC, it is referred to as indigenous plant and that its oil was used for lamps. Two varieties—the red and the white seeded—are mentioned. The oil was, and is still, used extensively in local medicines mainly as a laxative, but also to soften dry and coarse skin. The Chinese have used the oil for medicinal purposes, for centuries.

The castor plant appears to have originated in eastern Africa, especially around Ethiopia. It now grows throughout the warm-temperate and tropical regions and flourishes under a variety of climatic conditions. It can be grown almost anywhere and this is one of castor's greatest virtues.

The seeds of the plant contain alkoloid ricinine and toxalbumine ricin. They yield a fixed oil, which is used chiefly for medicinal purposes. Though castor plant or its oil is not a food, yet it is one of the most commonly used oils all over the world as a safe purgative and drug for reducing irritation of the skin and alleviating swelling and pain.

Castor oil chiefly consists of ricinoleate of glycerol or triricinolein with a small quantity of palmitin and stearin. Unlike most fixed oils, castor oil possesses the remarkable property of mixing with absolute alcohol and glacial acetic acid in all proportions. The glycerides of ricinoleic acid in castor oil are mainly responsible for its purgative effect.

Healing Power and Curative Properties

Castor is used very effectively in the treatment of rheumatic and skin disorders. It is a harmless purgative.

Rheumatism

A poultice of castor seeds can be applied with beneficial results to gouty and rheumatic swellings. A decoction of the roots of castor plant with carbonate of potash is useful in the treatment of lumbago, rheumatism and sciatica. A paste of the kernel without the embryo, boiled in milk, is also given as a medicine in these conditions.

Skin Disorders

A poultice of castor leaves is useful as an external application to boils and swellings. Coated with some bland oil such as coconut oil and heated, the hot leaves can be applied over guinea-worm sores to extract the worms. A poultice of castor seeds is also applied to scrofulous sores and boils due to tuberculosis of lymph nodes.

Problem of Breast Milk Secretion

Castor oil massaged over the breast after child-birth increases the flow of milk, as it stimulates the mammary glands. Castor leaves can also be used to foment the breasts, for the same purpose.

Dandruff

If used regularly as hair oil, it helps the growth of the hair and cures dandruff.

Constipation

Castor oil is a simple, harmless purgative and can be used without any rigid consideration and limitation of weather and the physiological nature of the patient. Generally, spring is the best season to administer purgatives, but castor oil, can safely be used round the year. It simply passes out after completing its purgative action, making the patient feel a mild irritation in the anus at that time.

Administration of castor oil as a purgative is very simple. About 30 to 60 grams of pure odourless castor oil is given orally with 250 to 375 grams of lukewarm milk. It acts just after an hour.

Those who find its use nauseating and unpalatable, can take it with ginger water or *aqua anisi* in place of milk. This greatly reduces its unpleasantness, while destroying mucous and promoting healthy appetite.

Other Uses

Natural Birth-Control: According to Ayurvedic and Unani treatises, if a woman chews one castor seed daily for a period of seven days after the menstruation she becomes sterile. This has been interpreted by many that castor seed is a herb for birth control[1] and if the woman swallows one castor seed, after the menstrual cycle she will not conceive during that month. When pregnancy is desired, the practice can be given up and conception follows after a year.

Castor oil massaged over the body, before bath, keeps the skin healthy and imparts sound sleep. Such an oil bath may be taken once in a week. Applying castor oil over hand and feet before going to bed keeps them soft and similarly over the eyebrows and eyelashes keeps them well-groomed.

---

1. Dr. Ganapathi Singh Verma, Miracles of Indian Herbs, p. 116.

Precautions: Repeated use of castor oil as a laxative should be avoided as it causes secondary constipation, that is, recurrence of the condition after cure. Persons suffering from kidney infections should not take castor oil as a purgative. It should also not be used when there is abdominal pain or intestinal infections such as appendicitis, enteritis or inflammation of the small intestine and peritonitis. Large doses of castor oil during the early months of pregnancy may cause abortion.

Celery

Botanical Name: *Apium graveolens*
Indian Name: *Ajmod or Ajwain-ka-patta*

Origin, Distribution and Composition

Celery is an important salad plant, consisting of the bulbous roots, green leaves and the stem. The leaves sprout directly from the fleshy roots. They are compound with long stalk; which are big and succulent. The fruits are small in size, dark brown in colour and have a peculiar flavour when cut open. The seeds are brown in colour.

In India, the leaves are not so popular, but, the root and the seeds are commonly used in Unani and Ayurvedic medicine.

Celery has been in cultivation for more than 2,000 years. It was known to the Chinese from the fifth century B.C. In England, where it grew wild, it was known as *smallage* and used in medicines. In the 16th and 17th centuries, it was brought into gardens and grown first as a medicinal plant and later as a flavouring for soups and stews.

Celery is a native of Europe and Asia. It is now grown widely in temperate regions and in tropical mountains. In India, large areas in the Punjab and Uttar Pradesh are given to the cultivation of celery for the production of the seed. It grows best with relatively cool weather and moderate rainfall during the crop season, at over 900 metres. As a salad crop, it is also grown in kitchen or home gardens.

Celery is an excellent basic food. It is one of the best sources of mineral salts and vitamins. An analysis of celery leaves shows them to consist of moisture 88.0 per cent, protein 6.3 per cent, fat 0.6 per cent, minerals 2.1 per cent, fibre 1.4 per cent and carbohydrates 1.6 per cent per 100 grams. Its mineral and vitamin contents are calcium, phosphorus, iron, carotene, riboflavin, niacine and vitamin C. Its calorific value is 37.

The fruits yield a volatile oil, pale yellow in colour. It consists of limonene d-selinene sedanonic acid, anhydride and sedanolide.

Healing Power and Curative Properties

The word celery is derived from Latin, *celeri* which means quick acting, and presumably refers to its therapeutic properties. The green leaves and stem of the bulbous root are all extremely rich in active ingredients that make celery an important medicinal plant. It has a well-balanced content of the basic minerals, vitamins and nutrients, besides a good concentration of plant hormones and essential oils that give celery its strong and characteristic smell. These oils have a specific effect on the regulation of the nervous system with their tranquilising properties. The seeds of celery relieve flatulence, increase the secretion and discharge of urine and act as an aphrodisiac. They are tonic, laxative and stimulant. They correct spasmodic disorders and can be used for aborting unwanted pregnancies.

Arthritis

Celery is useful in the treatment of arthritis due to its high sodium content. Its organic sodium tends to prevent and relieve the arthritic joint deposits by keeping lime and magnesia in a solution form. For optimum results, it should be taken in the form of freshly extracted juice, using its leaves as well as the stem.

Rheumatism and Gout

The alkaline elements in celery outweigh the acidic ones. It is therefore, very effective in diseases arising from acidity and toxemia, rheumatism and gout. A fluid extract of the seeds is more powerful than the raw vegetable.

Nervous Afflictions

An abundant use of celery juice combined with carrot juice is beneficial in the treatment of nervous afflictions resulting from the degeneration of sheathing or the protective cover of the nerves. It helps to restore these to their normal conditions therby alleviating the affliction.

Blood Disorders

The herb is valuable in diseases of the blood such as anaemia, leukaemia, Hodgkin's disease, purpura and haemophilia caused by the inorganic mineral elements and salts taken into the body by means of devitalized foods and sedatives. This plant is very high in magnesium and iron content, a combination which is invaluable as a food for the blood cells. The juice of celery in combination with carrot juice should be taken in the treatment of these disorders.

Respiratory Disorders

Celery is known to have antispasmodic properties and is useful in the treatment of asthma, bronchitis, pleurisy and tuberculosis. Its seeds serve the same purpose in such diseases.

Indigestion

The seeds of celery are an effective remedy for indigestion. A teaspoon of the seeds soaked in a glass of buttermilk for 5 to 6 hours should be ground in the same buttermilk mixture and administered to relieve indigestion

Kidney and Gall Stones

Celery is a valuable food for those who are prone to stone formation in the gall bladder or kidneys. Its regular use prevents stone formation.

General Debility

The powder of the dried root of the herb is an effective tonic in general debility or weakness and malnutrition. One teaspoon of this powder mixed with a tablespoon of honey is taken twice daily in such conditions.

Insomnia

Celery is also useful in the treatment of sleeplessness. Celery juice mixed with a tablespoon of honey makes a delightful drink. This mixture taken at night before retiring, will help one relax into a soothing and restful sleep.

Precautions: Celery with thick ribs and crisply brittle stalks should be selected for use. Its green portions should never be discarded or scraped, as by doing so, valuable vitamins are lost.

Other Uses

Celery can be eaten either raw in salads or in the cooked form. Soups and juices can also be prepared. In salads, it is usually taken with other vegetables and fruits. Cooked celery is delicious when taken with cream or butter. It is also used to flavour stews and sauces.

Chebulic Myroblan

Botanical Name: *Terminalia chebula retz*
Indian Name: *Harad or Haritaki*

Origin, Distribution and Composition

Chebulic myroblan is a wonderful herb and is known as long-life elixir. It is the fruit of a middle-sized or large tree which has egg-shaped 10 to 20 cm long leaves and dull white flowers in spikes at the end of its branches. The fruit, which is 2 to 4 cm long, has five distinct ribs on its body.

Chebulic myroblan is indigenous to India. It has been used in Indian system of medicine for a very long time. The physicians in ancient India used it in the treatment of diarrhoea, dysentery, heart-burn, flatulence, dyspepsia and liver and spleen disorders. There is an old Indian proverb which says, "If one bites a piece of *haritaki* everyday after meals and swallows its juice, he will remain free from all diseases."

The fruit of chebulic myroblan contains an astringent substance. The astringency is due to the characteristic principle chebulinic acid. It also contains tannic acid, gallic acid, resin and some purgative principle of the nature of anthraquinone.

Healing Power and Curative Properties

Among its many medicinal virtues, is its use as a mild, safe and efficacious laxative. The drug helps arrest secretion or bleeding and strengthens the stomach and promotes its action. It is useful in correcting disordered processes of nutrition by which the organism ingests, digests, absorbs, utilises and excretes food substance and restores the normal function of the system. This herb is one of the ingredients of the famous Ayurvedic preparation *triphala* which is used in the treatment of enlarged liver, stomach disorders and pain in the eyes.

Acidity

The juice of chebulic myroblan is highly beneficial in the treatment of acidity and heart-burn. It neutralizes the acidity in the stomach, if taken after meals. For better results, this juice should be combined with the juice of Indian gooseberry (amla). Chewing a piece of chebulic myroblan is an age-old remedy for heart-burn.

Asthma

A piece of the fruit chewed every night, will reduce asthmatic tendencies to the minimum.

Constipation

As a mild laxative, chebulic myroblan is useful in constipation. Either the pulp of 2 or 3 fruits with a little rock salt or a decoction of 6 fruits and 4 grams of cloves or cinnamon, should be taken daily at bed time to relieve constipation.

Diarrhoea and Dysentery

This herb is also an effective remedy for chronic diarrhoea and dysentery. Four grams of the pulp of the unripe fruit is given with honey and aromatics such as clove and cinnamon twice a day in the treatment of these diseases.

Piles

Chebulic myroblan is a popular remedy for piles. The fresh fruits should be fried to a golden brown colour in castor oil, powdered and stored. Half a teaspoon of this dissolved on the tongue at bedtime brings about normal bowel movement in the morning and its astringent property heals the pile masses.

Oral Inflammation

The use of a diluted decoction of chebulic myroblan is a popular gargle for mouth inflammation. The paste of the fruit mixed in thin buttermilk also makes a very effective gargle in gum inflammation. The powder of the fruit when applied directly on the painful tooth gives relief.

Skin Disorders

The herb is very useful in skin disorders like chronic ulcers, wounds and scalds. A fine powder of the fruit mixed with carrion oil—made from fat of an animal—makes an excellent ointment for burns and scalds.

Whitlow

Chebulic myroblan is also used to cure whitlow. The fruits are roasted, powdered and sieved. This powder is mixed in dilute tamarind water to make a fine paste which is applied on the infected finger. The astringent action of chebulic myroblan combines with the acidic effect of tamarind water to dry up infection.

Eye Disorders

A dilute decoction of chebulic myroblan used as an eye wash helps to relieve eye congestion. The fruit being astringent, decreases swelling and inflammation.

Mumps

A thick paste of chebulic myroblan applied over the swelling is a good remedy for treating mumps.

Vaginitis

A decoction of the herb is useful in vaginal irritation and inflammation. It should be used as a douche to wash the vulval parts. When there is thick white discharge, washing the part with a decoction made with neem leaves and chebulic myroblan fruits will help greatly.

Precautions: The use of chebulic myroblan should be avoided during pregnancy as it may cause abortion.

Other Uses

Hair Tonic: The herb is useful as a hair tonic. A paste of the fruit is boiled in coconut oil till its essence completely dissolves in the oil. This oil used regularly gives vitality to hair. Cheublic myroblan docoction is a popular hair rinse which many Indian women use to blacken grey hair.

Sweets and pickles based on chebulic myroblan are commonly used in Indian homes. They are believed to be digestive and mild laxative.

Chicory

Botanical Name: *Chichorium intybus*
Indian Name: *Kasni*

Origin, Distribution and Composition

Chicory, or endive, is a perennial herb with a long tap root. It has condensed, round stems, numerous light or dark green leaves and pale blue flowers. The leaves have a bitter taste; flowers open at sunrise and close at dusk.

Chicory is native to the Mediterranean region or, possibly, eastern India. It was known to the ancient Greeks and Romans and was cultivated in Egypt over 2000 years ago. The ancient physicians employed the plant in the treatment of several ailments. Classical writers like Horace, Virgil, Ovid and Pliny mentioned its use as a vegetable and a salad ingredient. Some scholars thought that the name succory came from the latin *succurrene* —which means to run under—because of the deep roots[1]. Another suggestion is that succory may be a corruption of chicory, or cichorium, a word of Egyptian origin. Chicory has been mentioned as a special skin nourisher by ancient herbalists. A tea made from the pale blue flowers of this plant was said to give glowing skin.

An analysis of chicory or endive leaves shows them to consist of 93.0 per cent moisture, 1.7 per cent protein, 0.1 per cent fat, 0.9 per cent fibre and 4.3 per cent carbohydrate per 100 grams. Its mineral and vitamin contents are calcium, phosphorus, iron, carotene, thiamine, riboflavin, niacin and vitamin C. Its calorific value is 20.

Chicory flowers contain a glucoside chichorin and bitter substances, lactucin and intbin. Seeds contain a bland oil and roots contain nitrate and sulphate of potash, mucilage and some bitter principle.

Healing Power and Curative Properties

Chicory is a tonic herb when taken in moderate quantitites. It increases the secretion and discharge of urine. It is also a

---

1. Rosemary Hemphilt, Herbs for all Seasons, p. 165, Penguin Books, England, 1975.

stimulant and a mild laxative. This herb helps the functions of the liver and gall bladder.

Eye Defects

Chicory contains food elements which are constantly needed by the optic system. It is one of the richest sources of vitamin A which is very useful for the eyes. The addition of juices of carrot, celery and parsley to chicory juice makes it a highly nourishing food for the optic nerve and the muscular system. It can bring amazing results in correcting eye defects. Half a litre to one litre daily of this combination has frequently corrected eye troubles within a few months, to the extent that normal vision was regained, making the use of glasses unnecessary.

Constipation

The herb is a natural laxative. It is, therefore, beneficial in the treatment of chronic constipation.

Anaemia

The herb, in combination with celery and parsley, is very helpful in anaemia. It is an effective blood tonic.

Liver and Gall Bladder Dysfunctions

Chicory flowers, seeds and roots are medicinally used in the treatment of liver disorders. About 30 to 60 ml of decoction of the flowers, seeds or roots can be used three times daily, with beneficial results, in the treatment of torpidity or sluggishness of the liver, biliary stasis or, stoppage of bile, jaundice and enlargement of the spleen. Endive or chicory juice, in almost any combination, promotes the secretion of bile and is, therefore, very good for both liver and gall bladder dysfunctions.

Respiratory Disorders

The combined juices of chicory, carrot and celery are most helpful in asthma and hay fever, provided milk and foods containing concentrated starches and sugars such as white rice, white flours, macaroni, sweets, pastries and cakes are eliminated from the diet. Powder of the dry root in doses of half a teaspoon, mixed with honey if taken thrice daily, is a good expectorant in chronic bronchitis.

Obstructed Menstruation

A decoction of chicory seeds is useful in treating obstructed menstruation.

Other Uses

The young leaves, preferably blanched, are eaten in salads. They may be mixed with other greens to minimise their strong flavour. The mature green leaves are sometimes used as a cooked vegetable. The root, when roasted and ground, is often used as an ingredient to mix with coffee, or is taken as a beverage on its own.

Cinnamon

Botanical Name: *Cinnamomum zeylanicum*
Indian Name: *Dalchini*

Origin, Distribution and Composition

Cinnamon is an evergreen tree which is small and bushy. Dried leaves of cinnamon, along with its dried inner bark are used all over the world as a spice or condiment. It has a pleasing fragrance and a warm, sweet and aromatic taste.

The bark of the tree is thick, smooth and light or dark brownish in colour. The inner bark is obtained from carefully selected shoots. It is then cured and dried. While drying, the bark shrinks and curls into a cylinder or quill.

Cinnamon tree was known to ancient physicians even before 2700 BC. The Chinese used the bark of this tree as a medicine. The Romans also knew about the medicinal value of this bark. Eminent physicians like Galen, Dioscoredes and Sasaferes described various uses of cinnamon. Indians knew about the therapeutic uses of this herb before the 8th century. The oldest record available about the description of cinnamon is in the *Torah*, the Jewish religious text. It was, however, Khizvenee who was the first person to give details about the medicinal virtues of this herb in the 13th century.

Cinnamon is a native of Sri Lanka and tropical Asia. It has been cultivated from ancient times. It appears to have reached Egypt and Europe by the fifth century BC. This tree occurs in South India upto altitudes of 500 metres but is more common at lower altitudes, even below 200 metres.

An analysis of cinnamon shows it to consist of moisture, protein, fat, fibre, carbohydrates and ash, besides calcium, phosphorus, iron, sodium, potassium, thiamine, riboflavin, niacin, vitamins C and A. Its calorific value is 355.

Cinnamon also contains an essential oil known as cinnamon oil. This oil consists of substantial amount of eugenol. The bark and green leaves also contain oil. The root bark oil differs from both stem bark and leaf oils.

Healing Power and Curative Properties

Cinnamon leaves are used in the form of powder or decoction. They are stimulant and useful in relieving flatulence and in increasing secretion and discharge of urine. Cinnamon prevents nervous tension, improves complexion and memory. A pinch of cinnamon powder mixed with honey does the trick if taken regularly every night for these purposes.

Common Cold

Cinnamon is an effective remedy for common cold. Coarsely powdered and boiled in a glass of water with a pinch of pepper powder and honey, it can be beneficially used as medicine in cases of influenza, sore throat, and malaria. Its regular use during the rainy season prevents attacks of influenza. Cinnamon oil, mixed with honey, gives relief from cold.

Digestive Disorders

Cinnamon checks nausea, vomiting and diarrhoea. It stimulates digestion. A tablespoon of cinnamon water, prepared as for cold and taken half an hour after meals, relieves flatulence and indigestion.

Bad breath

Cinnamon serves as a good mouth freshener.

Headache

Headache produced by exposure to cold air is readily cured by applying a paste of finely powdered cinnamon mixed in water on the temples and forehead.

Acne

Paste of cinnamon powder prepared with a few drops of fresh lime juice can be applied over pimples and blackheads with beneficial results.

Other Diseases

Cinnamon is highly beneficial in the treatment of several

other ailments, including spasmodic afflictions, asthma, paralysis, excessive menstruation, uterus disorders and gonnorhoea. It is sometimes used as a prophylactic agent, to control German measles.

Other Uses

Natural Birth-Control: Cinnamon can be used for natural birth-control. It has the remarkable effect of checking the early release of ova after child-birth. A piece of cinnamon taken every night for a month after child-birth delays menstruation for more than 15 to 20 months thus preventing early conception. It indirectly helps the secretion of breast milk. Prolonged breast feeding checks the restarting of menstruation after child-birth, according to studies.

Dried cinnamon leaves and inner bark are used for flavouring cakes and sweets and in curry powder. They are also used in incense, dentifrices and perfumes. Cinnamon bark oil is used for flavouring confectionery and liqueurs. It is also used in pharmaceutical and dental preparations. Cinnamon leaf oil is used in perfumes and flavourings as also in the synthesis of vanillin.

Clove

Botanical Name: *Syzygium aromaticum*
Indian Name: *Laung*

Origin, Distribution and Composition

Clove is the dried unopened flower bud obtained from a handsome, middle-sized, evergreen tree. The tree has a straight trunk and grows upto a height of 10 to 12 metres.

The clove has been used in India and China, for over 2,000 years, as a spice to check both tooth decay and counter halitosis, that is bad breath. In Persia and China, it was considered to have aphrodisiac properties.

The clove tree is a native of the Molucca islands. The Chinese obtained this spice by the 3rd century BC. Cloves were imported into Alexandria as early as 176 AD. By the fourth century AD it was well known in the Mediterranean and by the

69

8th century, throughout Europe. Today Zanzibar is the leading producer of cloves.

An analysis of clove shows it to consist of carbohydrates moisture, protein, volatile oil, non-volatile ether extract (fat), and crude fibre besides mineral matter, ash insoluble in hydrocloric acid, calcium, phosphorus, iron, sodium, potassium, thiamine, riboflavin, niacin, vitamins C and A. Its calorific value is 430.

The clove buds, stem and leaves, on steam distillation, yield a substantial amount of essential oil. The clove bud oil, derived from the dried buds by steam distillation, contains free eugenol, eugenol acetate and caryophyllene. The stem oil contains more free eugenal than the bud oil, besides eugenol acetate, in small quantity. The leaf oil contains much less of total eugenol than the bud oil and a very small quantity of eugenol acetate.

Healing Power and Curative Properties

Cloves have many medicinal virtues. They are stimulant. They are useful in counteracting spasmodic disorders and in relieving flatulence. They help stimulate sluggish circulation and thereby promote digestion and metabolism. In the Indian system of medicine, cloves are used in various conditions either in the form of a powder or a decoction made from them. Clove oil contains ingredients that help stabilize blood circulation and regulate body temperature. Clove oil, applied outwardly, has stimulating effects on the skin, producing heat and redness.

Digestive Disorders

Cloves promote enzymatic flow and boost digestive functioning. They are used in various forms of gastric irritability and dyspepsia. Licking the powder of fried cloves mixed with honey is effective in controlling vomiting. The anaesthetic action of clove numbs the gullet and stomach and stops vomiting.

Cholera

Cloves are very useful for treating cholera. About 4 grams of cloves are boiled in 3 litres of water until half the water has evaporated. This water, taken in draughts, will check severe symptoms of the disease.

Coughs

Chewing a clove with a crystal of common salt eases expectoration, relieves the irritation in the throat and stops cough in the pharyngitis—that is, inflammation of the pharynx. Chewing a burnt clove is also an effective medicine for coughs caused by congested throat and pharyngitis.

Three to five drops of clove oil mixed with honey and a clove of garlic helps alleviate the painful spasmodic coughs in tuberculosis, asthma and bronchitis. It should be taken once before going to bed.

Asthma
Clove is an effective remedy for asthma. A teaspoon of decoction prepared by boiling 6 cloves in 30 ml of water can be taken with honey thrice daily as an expectorant.

Teeth Disorders
The use of a clove in toothache decreases pain. It also helps to decrease infection due to its antiseptic properties. Clove oil, applied to a cavity in a decayed tooth, also relieves toothache.

Earache
A clove sauted in a teaspoon of sesame (til) oil and 3 to 5 drops of this (warm) oil put into the ear can cure earache.

Muscular Cramps
Muscular cramps are often relieved when the oil of clove is applied as a poultice near the affected portion.

Headaches
A paste of clove and salt crystals in milk is a common household remedy for headaches. Salt, as a hygroscopic agent, absorbs fluid and decreases tension.

Stye
Clove is one of the best remedies for styes which is an inflammation around the eyelash. A clove stub rubbed in water and then applied over the stye gives relief.

Other Uses
Cloves are used as a table spice and mixed with chillies, cinnamon, turmeric and other spices in the preparation of curry powder. They are also used to flavour the betel quid (pan pati). Clove oil is used in the manufacture of perfumes, soaps, bath salts and as a flavouring agent in medicine and dentistry.

Coriander

Botanical Name: *Coriandrum sativum*
Indian Name: *Dhania*

Origin, Distribution and Composition

Coriander is both an annual and a perennial herb. It is erect, sweet smelling and grows up to 20 cms in length with many branches. The stem is feeble, smooth and light green in colour. Leaves are compound, thin, alternate and easily breakable. Fruits are spherical–about one centimetre in diameter with some longitudinal ridges. They are green when tender and brownish yellow when ripe. They have a sweet fragrance.

Coriander is a native of the Mediterranean region, where it has been grown since ancient times. It is extensively cultivated in Europe, North Africa, India, South America, Malaysia, Thailand and China. It thrives in black soil and arid regions.

Coriander is rich in various food elements. An analysis of coriander leaves shows them to contain moisture 86.3 per cent, protein 3.3 per cent, fat 0.6 per cent, minerals 2.3 per cent, fibre 1.2 per cent and carbohydrates 6.3 per cent per 100 grams. The mineral and vitamin contents include calcium, phosphorus, iron, carotene, thiamine, riboflavin, niacin and vitamin C. They also contain sodium, potassium and oxalic acid. Their calorific value is 44.

Coriander seeds are dried when they are ripe. They have an aromatic odour and agreeable spicy taste. An analysis of the seeds shows them to contain moisture 11.2 per cent, protein 14.1 per cent, fat 16.1 per cent, minerals 4.4 per cent, fibre 32.6 per cent and carbohydrates 21.6 per cent per 100 grams. Their mineral and vitamin contents include calcium, phosphorus, iron, carotene, thiamine, riboflavin, and niacin. Their calorific value is 288.

Indian coriander contains an essential oil which causes irritation when in contact with skin for a long time. Besides essential oil, the seeds also contain a fatty oil.

Healing Power and Curative Properties

The leaves of coriander are stimulant and tonic. They strengthen the stomach and promote its action, relieve flatulence, increase secretion and discharge of urine and reduce fever. They act as an aphrodisiac, help in the removal of catarrhal matter and phlegm from the bronchial tubes thereby counteracting any spasmodic disorders. Coriander seeds reduce fever and promote a feeling of coolness. Coriander juice is highly beneficial in deficiencies of vitamin A, B_1, B_2, C and iron.

Digestive Disorders

One or two teaspoons of coriander juice, added to fresh buttermilk, is highly beneficial in treating digestive disorders such as indigestion, nausea, dysentery, hepatitis and ulcerative colitis. It is also helpful in typhoid fever.

Dry coriander treats diarrhoea and chronic dysentery, as well as being useful in acidity. A chutney made from dry coriander, green chillies, grated coconut, ginger and black grapes without seeds is a remedy for abdominal pain due to indigestion.

Small Pox

One teaspoon fresh coriander juice, mixed with 1 or 2 seeds of banana, given once daily regularly, for a week is a very effective preventive measure against small pox. It is believed that putting fresh leaf juice in the eyes, during an attack of small pox, prevents eye damage.

High Cholesterol Levels

Regular drinking of coriander water helps lower blood cholesterol as it is a good diuretic and stimulates the kidneys. It is prepared by boiling dry seeds of coriander and straining the decoction after cooling.

Excessive Menstrual flow

Coriander seeds check excessive menstrual flow. Six grams of the seeds should be boiled in half a litre of water, till only half the water remains. Sugar should be added to it and taken when it is still warm. The patient gets relief after taking the medicine for 3 or 4 days.

Conjuctivitis

A decoction prepared from freshly dried coriander is an excellent eye-wash in conjuctivitis. It relieves burning and reduces pain and swelling.

Skin Disorders

A teaspoon of coriander juice, mixed with a pinch of turmeric powder, is an effective remedy for pimples, blackheads and dry skin. The mixture should be applied to the face, after washing it thoroughly, every night before retiring.

Precautions: Dry coriander should be sparingly used by persons suffering from bronchial asthma and chronic bronchitis.

Other Uses

The young plants of coriander are used in chutneys, sauces, curries and soups. The volatile oil in it is used for flavouring and in medicine. In the dried form, coriander is an important ingredient of curry powder and is also used in pickling spices, sausages, seasoning, confectionery and for flavouring spirits, particularly gin.

Cumin Seeds

Botanical Name: *Cuminum cyminum*
Indian Name: *Jeera*

Origin, Distribution and Composition

Cumin is an annual herb, with a smooth surface and long, slender root. It grows up to a height of 35 to 45 cm. It produces a stem with many branches which bear long, finely divided, deep green leaves and small flowers, white or rose in colour. The plant has aromatic seed-like fruit, commonly known as cumin seed. It is oval-shaped, approximately 6 mm long and light yellowish-brown in colour. It has a peculiar, strong and heavy odour. The dried seeds form an essential ingredient of curry powder.

Cumin is a native of Egypt, Syria, Turkey and the Eastern Mediterranean region. It was one of the commonest spices during the Middle Ages. It is now grown in south-eastern Europe, north Africa, India and China.

An analysis of cumin seeds shows them to consist of moisture 6.2 per cent, protein 17.7 per cent, fat 23.8 per cent, crude fibre 9.1 per cent, carbohydrates 35.5 per cent and mineral matter 7.7 per cent per 100 grams. Their mineral and vitamin contents are calcium, phosphorus, iron, sodium, potassium, thiamine, riboflavin, niacin, vitamins C and A. Their calorific value is 460.

The dried fruit is crushed and subjected to fractional or steam disstilation to yield a valuable volatile oil pale-yellow in colour, which turns dark on keeping. The cumin aldehyde present in the volatile oil is readily converted artificially into thymol.

Healing Power and Curative Properties

The fruit is a rich source of thymol. Thymol is used as an anthelmintic against hookworm infections and also as an antiseptic in many proporietary preparations. It is a stimulant, which increases the secretion and discharge of urine and relieves flatulence. It strengthens the functions of stomach and arrests any bleeding.

Digestive Disorders

Cumin seeds are very useful in digestive disorders like biliousness, morning sickness, indigestion, atonic dyspepsia, diarrhoea, malabsorption syndrome, and flatulent colic. One teaspoon of cumin seeds is boiled in a glass of water and the decoction mixed with one teaspoon of fresh coriander leaf juice and a pinch of salt. This decoction can be taken twice daily after meals as a medicine for diarrhoea.

Piles

Black cumin is beneficial in the treatment of piles. About 60 grams of the seeds, of which half should be roasted, should be ground together. Three grams of this flour should be taken with water.

Insomnia

Cumin is valuable in relieving sleeplessness. A teaspoon of the fried powder of cumin seeds mixed with the pulp of a ripe banana can be taken at night to induce sleep.

Renal Colic

Black cumin seeds mixed with caraway seeds and black salt is useful in renal colic. About 20 grams of cumin seeds, 12 grams of caraway seeds and 6 grams of black salt are ground together and mixed with a little vinegar. This mixture can be taken in doses of 3 grams every hour till relief is obtained.

Common Cold

Dilute cumin water is an antiseptic beverage and very useful in common cold and fevers. To prepare cumin water, a teaspoon of cumin is added to boiling water, which is allowed to simmer for a few seconds and set aside to cool. If the cold is associated with sore throat, a few small pieces of dry ginger should be added to the water. It soothes throat irritation.

Problem of Breast Milk Secretion

A decoction of cumin seeds mixed with milk and honey, taken once daily during the entire period of pregnancy, helps the healthy development of the foetus, eases child-birth and increases the secretion of breast milk.

Amnesia

Cumin seeds are valuable in amnesia or dullness of memory. Three grams of black cumin seeds are mixed with 12 grams of pure honey and licked to get rid of in this condition.

Boils

Black cumin ground in water is applied as a paste over the boils with beneficial results.

Scorpion Sting

Paste of the cumin seeds prepared with onion juice, applied over scorpion sting will retard the frequency of upbeats.

Other Uses

The cumin seed is extensively used in mixed spices and for flavouring curries, soups, sausages, bread and cakes. It is an ingredient of curry powder, pickles and chutneys. It is also used to some extent in Indian medicine as a carminative.

Curry Leaves

Botanical Name: *Murraya koenigi*
Indian Name: *Curry patta*

Origin, Distribution and Composition

Curry leaves are derived from a beautiful, aromatic and more or less deciduous shrub growing up to 0.9 metre, or a small downy tree, up to 6 metres in height and 15 to 40 cms in diameter. The leaves are slightly bitter and aromatic.

The curry tree is a native of India and Sri Lanka. It grows in all tropical zones and more so in rich soils. It is cultivated extensively for its aromatic leaves and ornamental value throughout India.

An analysis of curry leaves shows them to consist of moisture 66.3 per cent, protein 6.1 per cent, fat (ether extract) 1.0 per cent, carbohydrates 16.0 per cent, fibre 6.4 per cent and mineral matter 4.2 per cent per 100 grams. Their mineral and vitamin contents are calcium, phosphorus, iron, nicotinic acid and vitamin C.

Fresh leaves on steam distillation under pressure yield a volatile oil. Besides the oil, the leaves contain a residual glucoside named as koenigin.

Healing Power and Curative Properties

Curry leaves possess the qualities of a herbal tonic. They strengthen the functions of stomach and promote its action. They are also used as a mild laxative. The leaves may be taken mixed with other mild tasting herbs. The juice extracted from 15 grams of leaves may be taken with buttermilk.

Digestive Disorders

Fresh juice of curry leaves, with lime juice and sugar, is an effective medicine in the treatment of morning sickness, nausea and vomiting due to indigestion and excessive use of fats. One or two teaspoons of juice of these leaves mixed with a teaspoon of lime juice may be taken in these conditions. The curry leaves, ground to a fine paste and mixed with buttermilk, can also be taken on an empty stomach with beneficial results in case of stomach upsets.

Tender curry leaves are useful in diarrhoea, dysentery and piles. They should be taken, mixed with honey. The bark of the tree is also useful in bilious vomiting. A teaspoon of the powder or the decoction of the dry bark should be given with cold water in this condition.

Diabetes

Eating 10 fresh fully grown curry leaves every morning for three months is said to prevent diabetes due to heredity factors. It also cures diabetes due to obesity, as the leaves have weight reducing properties. As the weight drops, the diabetic patients stop passing sugar in urine.

Kidney Disorders

The root of the curry plant also has medicinal properties. The juice of the root can be taken to relieve pain associated with the kidneys.

Premature Greying of Hair

Liberal intake of curry leaves is considered beneficial in preventing premature greying of hair. These leaves have the property to nourish the hair roots. New hair roots that grow are healthier with normal pigment. The leaves can be used in the form of *chutney* or the juice may be squeezed and taken in buttermilk or *lassi*.

Burns and Bruises

Curry leaves can be effectively used to treat burns, bruises and skin eruptions. They should be applied as a poultice over the affected areas.

Eye Disorders

Fresh juice of curry leaves suffused in the eyes makes them look bright. It also prevents the early development of cataract.

Insect Bites

Fruits of the tree, which are berries, are edible. They are green when raw, but purple when ripe. Juice of these berries, mixed with equal proportion of lime-juice, is an effective fluid for external application in insect stings and bites of poisonous creatures.

Other Uses

Hair Tonic: When the leaves are boiled in coconut oil till they are reduced to a blackened residue, the oil forms an excellent hair tonic to stimulate hair growth and in retaining the natural pigmentation.

Curry leaves have been used for centuries in South India as a natural flavouring agent in *samber, rasam* and curries. Chutney can be made by mixing the leaves with coriander leaves, coconut scrapings and tomatoes.

The leaves, bark and the root of the curry plant are used in indigenous medicine as a tonic, stimulant and antiflatulent.

Dandelion

Botanical Name: *Taraxacum officinale*
Indian Name: *Kukraundha or Kanphool*

Origin, Distribution and Composition

Dandelion is a hardy perennial herb and a tasty salad vegetable. The flower stems of this plant grows up to a height of 30 cm. The sharply-toothed leaves form flat rosettes on the ground. The fleshy hollow stem carries a single bright yellow flower.

The common name dandelion comes from the French *dent de lion*, meaning lion's tooth and refers to the dentate leaf edges. However, some believe that the name is derived from the resemblance of the yellow flower petals to an heraldic lion's golden teeth. The name of the genus come from the Greek *taraxos* meaning disorders and *akos* meaning remedy, indicating the curative qualities of the herb.

A very common plant, dandelion grows wild almost everywhere. Dandelion is native to Europe. In India it is found throughout the Himalayas, from 300 to 5400 metres and in the Mishmi Hills.

Nutritionally, the dandelion has remarkable value. It contains almost as much iron as spinach, four times the vitamin A content of lettuce and is a very rich source of magnesium, potassium, vitamin C, calcium and sodium. An analysis of dandelion shows it to consist of protein, fat and carbohydrates. Its mineral and vitamin contents are calcium, phosphorus, iron, magnesium, sodium, potassium, thiamine, riboflavin, vitamins C and A. Its calorific value is 45.

Dandelion contains a bitter crystalline principle, taraxacin and a crystalline substance, taraxacerin. It also contains the phytosterols, taraxasterol and humotaraxasterol.

Healing Power and Curative Properties

One can find the significant medicinal values of Dandelion from the Arabian writings of the 10th century, Welsh manuscripts of the 13th century and English herbal literature of the 16th and 17th centuries. Thanks to the efforts of herbalists, its virtues are now well known and respected, both for its therapeutic properties and as an alternative to tea and coffee.

The entire plant is used by many herbalists, although the tea is usually brewed from its root, which are a tonic. It increases the secretion and discharge of urine and acts as a mild purgative.

Bone Disorders

The readily available organic magnesium in dandelion makes the juice of the leaves, with or without the roots, valuable for all bone disorders. It is often mixed with juices of the leaves of carrots and turnips for treating these disorders.

Liver and Gall Bladder Dysfunctions

Dandelion benefits both liver and gall bladder in their vital role of handling fats within the body and aiding the detoxifying role of the liver. It is, therefore, useful in the disorders of these organs. Combined with the juice of watercress and with a diet without meat or much sugar and starch, it helps to make the liver and the gall bladder normal, and exercises a beneficial effect upon the nervous system. Sufferers from hepatitis can greatly benefit from dandelion tea.

General Debility

Dandelion can be used as a general body tonic for its influence in supporting waste functions of bowels, bladder and skin, which are the hard-working eliminating organs of our body.

Urinary Disorders

Dandelion tea, made from the buds, flowers, fresh leaves or even blanched leaves, can be very useful in cases of urinary disorders. Its familiar names of 'piss-le-lit' and 'bed-wetter' point to its characteristic effect, that of increasing the flow of urine. It can be very helpful in cases of slow start to passing urine. It is, however, important with most urinary troubles to drink plenty of water or other harmless, non-alcoholic drinks so that there can be a free flow of urine.

Warts

Dandelion is useful in the treatment of warts. The milk from the cut end of dandelion should be put on the wart twice or thrice a day

Other Uses

Tender leaves of dandelion are used as a tasty salad vegetable. The leaves should be torn to pieces rather than cut to keep their pungent flavour. These can also be cooked in a little boiling water or in combination with spinach and cooked in the same way. A tasty and beneficial soup can be made with chopped dandelion leaves. The dried leaves are used for tea and as an ingredient in diet drinks. Dandelion coffee is made from its dried, roasted and ground roots. It is a natural beverage, without the harmful effects of the conventional tea and coffee.

Datura

Botanical Name: *Datura stramonium*
Indian Name: *Dhatura*

Origin, Distribution and Composition

Datura is a bushy plant growing upto one metre in height. It has large egg-shaped leaves, very large white flowers and egg-shaped fruits, covered with prickles. The dried leaves, top portion of the flower and seeds of the plant constitute the drug.

Datura is referred to in ancient Indian literature as *shivashekhera* because the flowers are believed to be associated with Lord Shiva. It was known to the ancient Hindu physicians. They regarded the drug as an intoxicant, with emetic, digestive and healing powers. Smoking of datura seeds as a treatment for asthma was known during the vedic period.

Datura is indigenous to India. The plant grows in temperate Himalayas upto 2500 metres and in the hilly belts of Central and Southern India.

The leaves of the plant contain alkaloids. The cultivated plants produce higher percentage of alkaloids. Seeds yield deploid I and tetraploid II besides alkaloids. Some amount of alkaloids are there in dried seeds and fruits.

Healing Power and Curative Properties

The dried leaves and seeds of datura are used in the British and the United States Pharmacopoeia as antispasmodic under critical conditions of asthma and whooping cough. Datura possesses properties analogous to those of belladonna. It counteracts spasmodic disorders and induces deep sleep.

Asthma

Datura is very useful in asthma, when the smoke from the

81

burning leaves is inhaled. The leaves rolled into cigarettes can be smoked to relieve asthmatic attacks.

Malaria

Datura fruit is a specific remedy for phlegmatic and bilious types of malarial fever. A desired quantity of the fruit should be placed in an earthen pot and covered with a plaster composed of cloth and clay. It should be parched in 10 to 12 grams of cowdung cakes. When the fire gets extinguished and the pot is cold, the burnt fruit should removed, powdered and kept safely in a phial for use in malarial fever.

Heart Disorders

The herb is valuable remedy for heart disorders. It relieves cardiac pains, distress, palpitation and aortic disorders.

Earache

The leaves of the herb are useful in the treatment of earache. About 125 grams each of the juice of datura leaves and sesame oil should be boiled in a tin vessel on gentle fire. When half of the juice has evaporated, seven leaves of gigantic swallow wort *(akh)* should be put in it after smearing them with oil and sprinkling with powdered salt.The leaves should be boiled till they begin to char. This oil is then filtered through a coarse cloth and preserved in a bottle. A few drops of this oil in the ear cure earache and suppurative conditions of the ear.

Impotency

Datura is useful in impotency. The seeds of 15 ripe fruits should be extracted and boiled in eight kilograms of cow's milk on gentle fire. This milk should then be made into curd in the usual way and churned the next morning to extract butter which is stored in a broad-mouthed bottle. This butter, massaged every morning and evening on the penis and the spine, will provide the desired effect. It is also used as an oral medicine. Four grains with betel leaf can be taken. The use of this butter both externally and internally in this way will gradually promote health and vigour and restore absolute fitness in the body.

Baldness

A preparation made from datura seeds with other ingredients is useful in patchy baldness. A paste made with datura seeds, liquorice, saffron and milk cream is heated in coconut oil thoroughly till the solid mass converts to a charred powder. The oil when applied on bald patches has the power to stimulate hair growth. As datura is poisonous, hands should be washed thoroughly after handling the oil. The mixture should not be used on the scalp of children.

Problem of Breast Milk Secretion

The herb is highly beneficial in checking secretion of breast milk. In case of an unfortunate death of a newly born baby, accumulation of milk in the breasts of the mother poses a problem, causing severe pain. In such a case, warmed leaves of the datura tied on the breasts will help dry the milk without any pain and difficulty. Just 2 or 3 applications will bring the desired results.

Precautions: The usual dose of datura is about 2 decigrams. In large doses, it may lead to dilation of the pupils and dryness of the mouth and throat.

Dill

Botanical Name: *Anethum Sowa*
Indian Name: *Sowa*

Origin, Distribution and Composition

Dill is an annual or biennial herb. It has a smooth surface, finely dissected leaves, small yellow flowers and elliptic, flattened fruits. The single stalks grow to a height of 1 metre.

Dill was known to the ancient Greeks and Romans. Greeks covered their heads with dill leaves to induce sleep. It was also considered a charm against witchcraft in the Middle Ages and was burned to get rid of thunderous clouds and sulphurous fumes.

Dill is native to the Mediteranean region, South Russia and Scandinavia. It has been in cultivation for more than 2,000 years and is now grown widely in Asia Minor, North Africa, India and in all other tropical countries.

An analysis of Indian dill shows it to consist of moisture, mineral matter and acid-insoluble ash. The seeds of the plant yield an essential oil known as dill oil. The roots also yield essential oil containing 95 per cent of a-b pinene. The herb yields essential oil with high proportion of terpenes.

Healing Power and Curative Properties

Dill leaves are stimulant. They are useful in increasing secretion and discharge of urine and in counteracting spasmodic disorders. They are a soothing medicine and help improve the functioning of the stomach.

Digestive Disorders

Eating cooked dill regularly aids digestion and prevents constipation. The herb is specially useful for children. One or two teaspoons of decoction of the fresh leaves given—mixed with each baby feed—will prevent digestive disorders in babies and help them sleep well.

Dill oil, obtained by the distillation of the seeds, is also an effective medicine for hyperacidity, flatulent colic, hiccup and diarrhoea due to indigestion. A drop of dill oil, mixed in a teaspoon of honey, should be licked immediately after meals. Similarly, if a drop of it is administered with castor oil to young children it may prevent griping pain in the abdomen and increase purgative action by relaxing the intestines.

Diarrhoea and Dysentery

Dill seeds yield a very powerful carminative oil. When these are sauted in *ghee* with fenugreek seeds in equal numbers, they will serve a specific medicine for diarrhoea and acute bacillary dysentery. For optimum results, roasted seeds are powdered and mixed with curd or buttermilk.

Respiratory Disorders

Dill seeds are effective in respiratory disorders like colds, influenza and bronchitis. About 60 grams of infusion of the seeds mixed with honey should be taken thrice daily in such disorders.

Menstrual Disorders

Dill is useful in stimulating and regulating menstrual flow. It is effective in spasmodic menstrual pain in young girls and absence of menstruation due to anaemia, exposure to cold and pregnancy. About 60 grams of a decoction of the fresh leaves, mixed with a teaspoon of parsley juice, can be taken thrice daily in the treatment of the above disorders.

Bad Breath

Dill seeds are highly useful in curing bad breath. The seeds are chewed for this purpose.

Boils and Swellings

A paste of fresh dill leaves can be applied as a poultice to ripen blood boils. Its application with a little turmeric powder (*haldi*) prevents any formation of pus in ulcers and heals them quickly. Leaves boiled in sesame (*til*) oil makes an excellent liniment for reducing swelling and pain of the joints.

Precautions: Dill leaves are slightly pungent, aromatic and bitter in taste. They should, therefore, be taken only in combination with other mild tasting leafy vegetables.

Other Uses

Pregnancy and Lactation: Dill is of great value to pregnant women and nursing mothers. Its regular use after childbirth increases the quantum of breast milk. It prevents any early ovulation thereby establishing as an effective birth control device.

The fresh green plant is used as a flavouring for soups, sauces and other culinary purposes. The seeds are used as a substitute for caraway seeds and as a source of dill-water, especially for relieving flatulence in babies. The leaves can serve as supplement to vegetable salads. The leaves and seeds can be used in making pickles or chutneys and summer beverages.

Ephedra

Botanical Name: *Ephedra gerardiana wall*
Indian Name: *Asmania*

Origin, Distribution and Composition

Ephedra is a small shrub about one metre high. It has many branched stems, straight branches and minute leaves, reduced to two-toothed sheaths or covering. The dried stems of ephedra, collected in autumn, constitute the drug. The trade name is based on its scientific name.

The Ayurvedic name of this herb is *somlata*. Many Ayurvedic physicians believe that ephedra is the same herb from which *somras* was prepared in the vedic age and which is widely mentioned in ancient ayurvedic texts like *Charaka Sushruta*. There is, however, no positive evidence to justify such belief.

The ephedra is indigenous to India and contains alkaloids. The principal alkaloid is ephedrine which is similar to adrenaline in pharmacological action. The other alkaloid contained in the herb is pseudo-ephedrine.

Healing Power and Curative Properties

No drug of recent years has attracted so much attention from the medical profession as ephedrine, an extract prepared from the herb ephedra, by allopathic pharmacists. It has earned a great reputation as an instantaneous cure for asthma and some other diseases. Ayurvedic physicians, however, maintain that the use of the herb in the original form is safer than ephedrine.

Asthma

The main use of ephedra is in the treatment of asthma, particularly bronchial asthma. The powder of the herb in doses ranging from 0.5 to 2.0 grams should be swallowed with water in such symptoms. It will give immediate relief by facilitating unrestricted discharge of the accumulated phlegm and clearance of the air passage, followed by restful sleep.

Rheumatism

The powder as well as infusion of ephedra is useful in acute rheumatism. Its use for 10 to 12 days consecutively will relieve painful, inflamed joints and leave the patient healthy. It, however, is not of much value in chronic cases. Ephedra stands as an infallible remedy for rheumatic troubles where allopathic medicines like salicylate of soda, aspirin and antipyrin fail to produce any visible result. At the same time, it does not produce any side-effects on the heart. It is a good stimulant for cardiac results.

Heart Disorders

Ephedra is an excellent stimulant for the heart. It has proved very effective especially in cases where the heart is affected by infections of pneumonia and diptheria.

Urinary Disorders

Ephedra has some effect on the urinary bladder. It has proved especially useful in controlling night wetting in children.

Other Disorders

Ephedra has been used successfully in several other disorders like hay-fever and rashes of allergic origin. Several preparations based on ephedrine are being used today in medicine. These include nasal sprays used in sinusitis, asthmatic attacks and inflammation of the mucous membrane.

Precautions: The use of ephedra in large doses should be avoided as it may lead to nausea, sweating or certain skin ailments.

Methods for Use: The herb can be taken either in the form of powder or in the form of decoction. Its powder provides excellent results if given every morning and evening with water or honey. In case of decoction, about 12 grams of crushed ephedra plant should be put in a litre of water and evaporated to 500 ml. The decoction should then be strained and preserved in a tightly corked bottle for use when needed. It should be administered in 30 ml dose daily.

Fenugreek

Botanical Name: *Trigonella foenum graecum*
Indian Name: *Methi*

Origin, Distribution and Composition

Fenugreek is an erect, strongly scented, robust, annual herb, about 30 to 80 cms high. It has compound leaves of light green colour, 2 to 2.5 cms long, yellow flowers and thin pointed pods. The seeds are brownish-yellow and have a peculiar odour.

Fenugreek is a native of Eastern Europe and Ethiopia. It has been used since ancient times both as a food and medicine by the people living on the shores of the Mediterranean and across Asia.

The leaves contain moisture 86.1 per cent, protein 4.4 per cent, fat 0.9 per cent, minerals 1.5 per cent, fibre 1.1 per cent and carbohydrates 6.0 per cent per 100 grams of edible portion. Its mineral and vitamin contents are calcium, phosphorus, iron, carotene, thiamine, riboflavin, niacin and vitamin C. Its calorific value is 49.

Fenugreek seeds contain moisture 13.7 per cent, protein

26.2 per cent, fat 5.8 per cent, minerals 3.0 per cent, fibre 7.2 per cent and carbohydrates 44.1 per cent per 100 grams. Their mineral and vitamin contents are calcium, phosphorus, carotene, thiamine, riboflavin and niacin. Several alkaloids have been found in fenugreek seeds. Its calorific value is 333.

The seeds contain alkaloid trigonelline and choline, essential oil and saponin. Trigonelline has highly toxic action on neuromuscular preparations. The seeds also contain fixed and volatile oil, mucilage, bitter extractive and a yellow colouring substance. Air-dried seeds contain a little amount of trigonelline and nicotinic acid.

Healing Power and Curative Properties

Fenugreek has excellent medicinal virtues. Its regular use helps keep the body clean and healthy. The leaves of fenugreek are aromatic, cooling and mild laxative. The seeds exercise soothing effect on the skin and mucous membranes, relieving any irritation of the skin and alleviating swelling and pain. They increase the secretion and discharge of urine, relieve flatulence and promote lactation in nursing mothers. They also arrest any secretion or bleeding and have an aphrodisiac effect. They are the best cleansers within the body, highly mucus-solvent and soothing agents.

Digestive Disorders

Fenugreek leaves are beneficial in the treatment of indigestion, flatulence and sluggish liver. Boiled and fried in butter, they alleviate biliousness. The seeds are also useful in the treatment of colic, flatulence, dysentery, diarrhoea and dyspepsia.

Anaemia

The leaves help in blood formation. The cooked leaves help prevent anaemia and run down condition in girls, usually associated with the onset of puberty and a sudden spurt in growth. The seeds also help in recovering from anaemia, being rich in iron.

Deadened Senses

The seeds help restore the deadened senses of taste or smell. The sense of taste dulls due to improper functioning of the salivary glands which often become clogged with mucus and accumulated juices, causing swelling. Similarly, the sense of smell is obstructed due to prolonged accumulations of mucus and other impurities in the nose where the olfactory nerves, that is, the special sensory nerve of smell are based.

Fevers

Tea made from fenugreek seeds is equal in value to quinine in reducing fevers. It is particularly valuable as a cleansing and soothing drink. Fenugreek seeds, when moistened with water become slightly mucilaginous, and hence the tea made from with them has the power to dissolve sticky substance like mucus.

Stomach Disorders

This tea soothes inflamed stomach and intestines, cleansing the stomach, bowels, kidneys and respiratory tract of excess mucus. It is beneficial in the healing of peptic ulcers, as the mild coating of mucilaginous matter deposited by fenugreek provides a protective layer for the ulcers, when it passes through the stomach and intestines.

Respiratory Infections

During the early stages of any of the respiratory tract infections, such as bronchitis, influenza, sinusitis, catarrh and suspected pneumonia, fenugreek tea helps the body to perspire, dispel toxicity and shorten the gestation period of fever. One can take upto 4 cups of the fenugreek tea. The quantity may be reduced as the condition improves. To improve flavour, a few drops of lemon juice can be used. During the treatment, no other food or nourishment should be taken, as fasting aids the body to correct these respiratory problems in a few days.

Bad Breath and Body Odour

The tea is also beneficial in bad breath and body odour. Unpleasant odours emanate from the body due to accumulations of hardened mucus and other toxins in the nasal and oral passages, the gastro-intestinal tract, the urinary tract, the blood and the vagina. Fenugreek tea, taken regularly helps remove these accumulations from these spots where mouthwash and soap can never penetrate.

According to Lelord Kordel, one of the world's most famous nutritionist, "So potent are the volatile oils in fenugreek and so thorough a job of cleansing do they perform, that often a decided fragrance of fenugreek seeds emanates from the body pores of a person using the herb regularly. These oils seek out and penetrate the most remote crevices and creases of the membranous linings within the body cavities. The volatile oils are absorbed into the cell tissues to do their job of rejuvenating our body. Some of them finally find their way into the sweat glands to cleanse and awaken any sluggishness in these parts."[1]

Diabetes

Fenugreek seeds can also be taken for diabetes. The normal dose is 2 teaspoons of powdered seeds taken daily in broth or milk. Two teaspoons of the seeds can also be swallowed whole, daily. Alternatively, they may be soaked in a cup of water at night and the water taken in the morning.

Dandruff

Fenugreek seeds are useful in the removal of dandruff. Two tablespoonfuls of the seeds are soaked overnight in water. In the morning, the softened seeds are ground into a fine paste and applied on the scalp and left on for half an hour. The hair is then washed thoroughly with soapnut (rita nut) solution or *shikakai*. A paste of the fresh leaves of fenugreek applied over the scalp regularly before washing the hair also cures dandruff.

Mouth Ulcers

The herb helps in the healing of mouth ulcers. An infusion of the leaves is used as a gargle for recurrent ulcers.

Sore throat

A gargle made from fenugreek seeds is best for ordinary sore throat. For the gargle, the solution should be much stronger than the tea. Two tablespoons of fenugreek seeds are put in a litre of water and allowed to simmer for half an hour over a low flame. It is cooled to room temperature and strained. The entire liquid is used as a gargle.

Leucorrhoea

Fenugreek tea used as a douche, is very effective in treating leucorrhoea. The solution is prepared in the same manner as for throat gargle.

---

1. Lelord Kordel, Health The Easy Way, p. 51, Award Books, New York, 1976.

Swellings

A poultice of the leaves can be applied with advantage in external and internal swellings. It is also useful in burns due to its cooling properties.

Other Uses

Beauty Aid: A paste of the fresh leaves applied over the scalp regularly before taking bath, helps hair grow. while preserving the natural colour and keeping the hair silky. The paste applied on the face every night before going to bed and washed with warm water, prevents one from getting pimples, blackheads, dryness of the face and early appearance of wrinkles. It also improves complexion and makes one look years younger.

Pregnancy and Lactation: The seeds fried in *ghee* are finely powdered, with wheat flour and sugar to prepare a *halwa*. Taken in small quantity daily, this helps in quick normalisation after delivery. The seeds, made into a gruel, and given to nursing mothers increases the flow of milk.

Steaming is considered the best method of cooking leaves; in this the vitamins are retained and the vegetable becomes palatable. The dried leaves can be compared to pulses for their protein content. They supplement the lysine-deficient cereal diets.

In Indian homes, fenugreek seeds are generally used as a condiment for flavouring. They form an ingredient of curry powder. They are also used in bread and bakery products in Egypt and Ethiopia. In Switzerland they are used for flavouring cheese. In the U.S.A. they are used in the preparation of spice blends and a wide variety of soups and stews. The seeds are used in the preparation of hair tonics and cosmetics in Java.

Garlic

Botanical Name: *Allium Sativum*
Indian Name: *Lahsoon*

Origin, Distribution and Composition

Garlic is an erect biennial herb of the onion family, normally grown as an annual. It has irregular roots, condensed, flattened stem and narrow, flat leaves. The bulb consists of 6 to 35 bulblets called cloves, enclosed in a thick whitish, glistening and transparent covering.

Garlic has been highly valued for centuries all over the world for its health-building qualities. Khnoum Khoufouf, the builder of one of the oldest pyramids, (4500 BC) was among the first to recognise the virtues of garlic, for he decreed that all his workers should take garlic every day to maintain their health and strength. Hippocrates, the father of medicine (460-357 BC) recommended the use of this herb in infectious diseases and particularly prescribed it for intestinal disorders.

Garlic is believed to have originated in Central Asia and was known to the Chinese as far back as 3,000 BC. It continues to be one of the staple spices of the Chinese diet till today. Egyptians, Greeks and Romans also used garlic both as a staple food and as a medicine for several ailments. It spread to all parts of the world and is now widely grown in the Mediterranean region, India, Philippines, China, Ethiopia, Kenya, Brazil and Mexico. It grows well in cool climates with dry weather.

An analysis of garlic shows it to contain moisture 62.0 per cent, protein 6.3 per cent, fat 0.1 per cent, minerals 1.0 per cent, fibre 0.8 per cent and carbohydrates 29.8 per cent per 100 grams of edible portion. Its mineral and vitamin contents are calcium, phosphorus, iron, thiamine, riboflavin, niacin and vitamin C. It also contains traces of iodine, sulphur and chlorine. Its calorific value is 145.

The bulbs yield an essential oil containing allyl propyl disulphide, diallyl disulphide and two other sulphur compounds. They also contain antiseptic and hypotensive, or, causing low blood pressure principles—allicin, allisatin I and allisatin II.

Healing Power and Curative Properties

In herbal medicine, garlic has been traditionally used for asthma, deafness, leprosy, bronchial congestion, arteriosclerosis —that is hardening of arteries—fevers, worms and liver and gall bladder trouble. Garlic is good for the heart, a food for the hair, a stimulant to appetite, a strength-giving food, useful in leucoderma, leprosy, piles, worms, catarrhal disorders, asthma and cough.

Clinical experiments in recent times have confirmed several ancient beliefs about the healing value of this herb. These experiments have in fact proven much greater power of garlic than known previously. The unpleasant odour in garlic is due to its sulphur content. This mineral is contained to a greater degree in its volatile oil, which has remarkable medicinal virtues.

Garlic juice has a most beneficial effect on the entire system. The ethers in garlic juice are so potent and penetrating, that they help dissolve accumulation of mucus in the sinus cavities, bronchial tubes and the lungs. They help in the expulsion of poisons from body through pores of the skin.

Chest Diseases

Garlic has proved effective in certain diseases of the chest. It reduces foetidity or stinking of the breath in pulmonary gangrene. Garlic is useful in the treatment of tuberculosis.

In *Ayurveda*, a decoction of garlic boiled in milk is considered a wonderful drug for tuberculosis. One gram of garlic, 250 ml of milk and a litre of water are boiled together till its reduces to one fourth of the decoction. It should be taken thrice a day. Taken in sufficient quantities, it is a marvelous remedy for pneumonia.

Asthma

Three cloves of garlic boiled in milk, can be used every night with excellent results in asthma. A pod of garlic is peeled, crushed and boiled in 120 ml pure malt-vinegar. It is strained after cooling and an equal quantity of honey is mixed and preserved in a clean bottle. One or two teaspoons of this syrup can be taken with fenugreek decoction in the evening and before retiring. This has been found effective in reducing the severity of asthmatic attacks.

Digestive Disorders

Garlic is one of the most beneficial herbs for the digestive system. It is good for the lymph, and aids elimination of noxious waste matter in the body. It stimulates peristaltis, or movement of the intestines—and the secretion of the digestive juices. Crushed cloves of garlic may be infused in water or milk and taken for all disorders of digestion. It has an antiseptic effect and is an excellent remedy for infectious diseases and inflammations of the stomach and intestine. Garlic oil is absorbed into the alimentary tract and is eliminated partly through the urine.

The herb is an excellent worm expeller. It is also good in

treating various forms of diarrhoea. Problems such as colitis, dysentry and many other intestinal disorders can be successfully treated with fresh garlic or garlic capsules. One garlic capsule taken thrice a day is usually sufficient to correct mild cases of diarrhoea or dysentery. For more persistent cases, upto 6 capsules a day can be taken. Garlic has the ability to destroy harmful bacteria in the intestines without affecting the beneficial organisms which aid digestion.

High Blood Pressure

Garlic is one of the most effective remedies for lowering blood pressure. Pressure and tension are reduced because it has the power to ease the spasm of the small arteries. It also slows the pulse and modifies the heart rhythm, besides relieving symptoms of dizziness, shortness of breath and formation of gas within the digestive tract. The average dosage should be 2 to 3 capsules a day to reduce the blood pressure.

Rheumatism

In Russia, garlic is used extensively in the treatment of rheumatism and associated diseases. Even in Britain, garlic is recommended for rheumatic afflictions. Recent experiments in Japan tested a garlic extract on patients with lumbago and arthritis with a large number being benefited without any undesirable side-effects. Its anti-inflammatory property accounts for its effectiveness in the treatment of arthritis and rheumatism.

Heart Attack

Following a recent study, a West German doctor claims that garlic may prevent heart attack. Garlic helps to break up cholesterol in the blood vessels, thereby preventing any hardening of arteries which leads to high blood pressure and heart attack. If a patient takes garlic after a heart attack, the cholesterol level comes down. Though the earlier damage may not be repaired, the chances of new attacks are reduced.

Cancer

Garlic preparations, including extracts and juices, have been used successfully against cancer in both animal and human studies[1]. A study report tells of mice being injected with cancer cells, some of which were treated with garlic extract and some were not. The mice not given garlic died within 16 days while the ones treated, lived for 6 months. In Russian studies, garlic preparations have been found to retard tumour growth not only in animals, but also in human beings, writes Dr. Airola.

Dr. Tariq Abdullah, a US researcher and staff physician of the Akbar clinic and Research Institute in Panama City, Florida, said recently that he and his colleagues found that white blood cells from six patients given garlic killed 139 per cent more tumour cells in a lab dish than did cells from people who did not eat garlic[2].

Whooping Cough

Garlic is an excellent remedy for whooping cough. Syrup of garlic should be taken in doses of five drops to a teaspoon, two or three times a day in treating this condition. It should be given more often if the coughing spells are frequent and violent.

Blood Disorders

The herb is regarded as a rejuvenator. It has been found to help remove toxins, revitalise the blood, stimulate circulation and promote intestinal flora, or colony of bacteria that prevent infection by harmful bacteria.

Skin Disorders

Garlic has been used successfully for a variety of skin disorders. Pimples disappear without a scar when rubbed with raw garlic several times a day. Even very persistent forms of acne, in some adults, have been healed with garlic. The external use of garlic helps to clear the skin of spots pimples and boils. The process is further helped by also taking the garlic internally to purify the blood. A regular course of three garlic capsules per day should help to clear minor skin infections quickly.

Garlic, rubbed over ringworm, gives quick relief. The area is burnt by the strong garlic and later the skin peels off and the ringworm is cured.

---

1. M. K. Kaul, *Mirror* (monthly magazine), p. 40, June issue, Bombay, 1986

2. PTI report, *Times of India*, 1987

Wounds and Ulcers

The herb has been used as an antiseptic in wounds and ulcerations with beneficial results. Garlic juice with three parts of distilled water is employed as a lotion for cleansing infected wounds. Definite improvement is noticed within 24 hours and substantial improvement within 48 hours. Application of dressing, containing 15 per cent garlic juice once a day over an ulcer removes pus in a few days. It also relieves pain within a short time. Russian physicians are making extensive use of garlic in the healing of wounds.

Diphtheria

Garlic is considered an excellent remedy for diphtheria. Chewing a clove of garlic cures the infected mucous membranes, reduces temperature and provides relief. About 30 to 60 grams of garlic can be used in this way in three or four hours for the membranes to disappear in a week. However, it is advisable to hospitalise and isolate the patient as soon as the diagnosis is confirmed.

Other Uses

Aphrodisiac Effect: Garlic has a pronounced aphrodisiac effect[1]. It is a tonic for the loss of sexual power from any cause. It also treats sexual debility and impotency caused by overindulgence in sex and nervous exhaustion from dissipating habit. It is said to be especially useful to old men with nervous tension and failing libido.

Garlic is the most widely used of the cultivated alliums after onions. It is used both as a food and seasoning, in the preparation of soups, sauces and pickles. In Spain and Italy, it is used with almost every food.

---

1. Dr. S.J. Singh, Food Remedies, 4th edition, p. 92, Nature Cure Council of Medical Research, Lucknow, 1982.

Ginger

Botanical Name: *Zingiber officinale*

Indian Name: *Adrak*

Origin, Distribution and Composition

Ginger is a perennial herb, with underground branching stems (rhizomes) which are swollen and tough. The leaves and rhizomes of ginger have a characteristic fragrance when cut or bruised. Rhizomes are dug out after the leafy parts are dried. The sun-dried ginger is known as *sounth* in Hindi.

There are numerous references to ginger in Sanskrit literature and in Chinese medical treatises. The Sanskrit name *Singabera* gave rise to the Greek Zingiberi and to the Latin Zingiber. Ginger has been used as a medicine in India from Vedic period and is called *maha-aushadhi*, meaning the great medicine. Ancient physicians used it as a carminative or anti-flatulent. Galen, the Greek physician, used ginger to rectify the defective humours or fluids of the body. He used ginger to treat paralysis caused by phlegmatic imbalance in the body. Aviceena used it as an aphrodisiac. Pomose also used ginger in the treatment of gout, centuries ago.

Ginger is believed to have originated in India and was introduced in China at a very early date. It appears to have been used as a spice and a medicine from early times by the Indians and the Chinese. It was known in Europe in the first century A.D. and was mentioned by Dioscoredes and Pliny.

An analysis of fresh ginger shows it to contain moisture 80.9 per cent, protein 2.3 per cent, fat 0.9 per cent, minerals 1.2 per cent, fibre 2.4 per cent and carbohydrates 12.3 per cent per 100 grams. Its mineral and vitamin contents are calcium, phosphours, iron, carotene, thiamine, riboflavin, niacin and vitamin C. Its calorific value is 67.

The composition of ginger varies with the type or variety, region, agro-climatic conditions, methods of curing, drying, packaging and storage. Chemical analysis of 26 varieties of ginger grown in India was conducted at CFTRI, Mysore, which showed the following important ingredients: volatile oil, oleoresin (acetone extract), water extract, cold alcohol extract, substantial amount of starch, total ash, water soluble ash, acid insoluble ash and alkalinity of ash of unpeeled ginger.

97

On steam distillation, dried, cracked and crushed ginger yields a pale yellow, viscid oil. The oil possesses the aromatic odour but not the pungent flavour of the spice. The odour of the oil is lingering.

Healing Power and Curative Properties

Ginger is widely used in local medicines in India and the Far East. Taken internally, it is a stimulating carminative and externally, it is used as a rubefacient that is, counter-irritant for relief of muscular pain. Like many other spices, ginger is believed to have aphrodisiac properties.

Digestive Disorders

Ginger is extremely useful in the treatment of dyspepsia, flatulence, colic, vomiting, spasms and other painful affections of the stomach and the bowels, not accompanied by fever. Chewing a piece of fresh ginger regularly after meals prevents these ailments. This protective action is due to the excessive secretion of saliva, diastase enzyme and volatile oil.

Half a teaspoon of fresh ginger juice, mixed with one teaspoon each of fresh lime and mint juices and a tablespoon of honey, constitutes an effective medicine for dyspepsia, nausea and vomiting due to biliousness, indigestion caused by intake of heavy non-vegetarian and fried fatty food, morning sickness, jaundice and piles. This mixture should be taken thrice daily in the treatment of these conditions.

Coughs and Cold

The herb is an excellent remedy for coughs and colds. Extracted juice of ginger with honey is taken three or four times a day in case of coughs. In case of colds, ginger cut into small pieces is boiled in a cup of water. After straining, with half-a-teaspoon of sugar, it should be taken hot. Ginger tea, prepared by adding a few pieces of ginger into boiled water before adding tea leaves, is another effective remedy for frequent colds and associated fevers.

Respiratory Disorders

A teaspoon of fresh ginger juice mixed with a cup of fenugreek decoction and honey to taste, makes an excellent diaphoretic mixture to proliferate sweating and reduces fever in influenza. It acts as an expectorant in bronchitis, asthma, whooping cough and tuberculosis of the lungs.

Impotency

Ginger juice is aphrodisiac. For better results, half a teaspoon of ginger juice honey with a half-boiled egg and is taken at night for a month. It tones up the sex organs and cures impotency, premature ejaculation and spermatorrhoea, or involuntary seminal discharge.

Menstrual Disorders

For menstrual disorders, a piece of fresh ginger is pounded and boiled in a cup of water for a few minutes. The infusion, sweetened with sugar, is taken thrice daily after meals for painful or irregular menstruation caused by exposure to cold winds or by cold bath.

Aches and Pains

Ginger is an excellent pain killer. It can cure all types of pain. In headache, ginger ointment made by rubbing dry ginger with a little water on a grinding stone and applied to the forehead affords relief. It allays toothache when applied to the gum. In case of earache, a few drops of ginger juice gives relief.

Other Uses

Ginger is available in two forms, fresh and dried. Both the forms are effective. As the taste of ginger is not very palatable, it is carefully adapted to the palate by putting it in vegetables. In western countries, it is widely used for culinary purposes in gingerbread, biscuits, cakes, puddings, soups and pickles. It is a common constituent of curry powder. Ginger is the most widely-used spice in Chinese cookery.

The essential oil from the rhizomes is used in the manufacture of flavouring essence and in perfumery. An oleoresin is also extracted, in which the full pungency of the spice is preserved; it is used for flavouring and medicinal purposes.

Henna

Botanical Name: *Lawsonia Inermis*
Indian Name: *Mehndi*

Origin, Distribution and Composition

Henna is a middle-sized shrub with many branches. It has small white or pinkish fragrant flowers in large terminal bunches, and small round fruits. The trade name henna is based on the word *hina* which is the Arabic name of the drug.

The plant occurs in several parts of India, chiefly in the drier parts of the peninsula, and is usually cultivated in hedges. It is also cultivated for commercial purposes in Punjab, Gujarat, Madhya Pradesh and Rajasthan.

The leaves contain a glucoside colouring matter and hennotanic acid. On petroleum ether extraction, the seeds of the plant yield a viscous oil containing behenic, arachidic, stearic, palmitic, oleic and linoleic acids.

Healing Power and Curative Properties

The leaves have medicinal properties like arresting secretion or bleeding and preventing skin diseases. The bark and seeds of the plant are used in Ayurvedic and Unani medicine.

Dysentery

The seeds of the henna plant are effective in the treatment of dysentery. They are powdered, mixed with *ghee* and made into small balls of the size of a betel nut. It is also very helpful in this condition, when taken with water.

Liver Disorders

The bark of the plant is effective in the treatment of liver disorders like jaundice and enlargement of the liver. Either its powder is used in 1.25 to 5 decigram doses or its decoction in 30 to 60 gram doses in the treatment of these disorders.

Baldness

Henna helps in the treatment of baldness. Mustard oil boiled with henna leaves, promotes healthy growth of hair. Two hundred and fifty grams of mustard oil is boiled in a tin basin. Sixty grams of the leaves are gradually added to the oil and heated. The oil is then filtered through a cloth and stored in a bottle. Regular massage with this oil produces abundant hair.

Prickly Heat

Henna leaves are beneficial in the treatment of prickly heat. The leaves ground with water are applied over the affected area.

Headaches

Henna flower cures headaches caused by the heat of the sun. The headache is relieved by a plaster made of henna flowers in vinegar and applied over the forehead.

Burning Sensation on the Feet

A paste of the leaves is applied on the soles relieves in this condition.

Skin Diseases

Henna leaves are effective in the treatment of skin problems like boils and burns. They are locally applied on the affected area. Bruised leaves can be applied beneficially in rheumatic joints, inflammatory swellings, bruises and leprosy.

Sore Throat

A decoction of the leaves can be used as gargle, with beneficial results, in case of sore throat.

Women's Ailments

Pessaries or vaginal suppositories made of the leaves and seeds can be used beneficially in the treatment of excessive menstruation, vaginal discharges and leucorrhoea, or excessive white discharge.

Other Uses

Spermatorrhoea or Involuntary Ejaculation: The juice of fresh leaves is beneficial, provided it is given in doses of 8 to 16 grams.

Henna is mainly used as a colouring agent. It is mixed with other natural dyes and is largely used as hair dye and even for textiles. The oil obtained from its flowers is used in perfumery.

Hog Weed

Botanical Name: *Boerhaavia diffusa*
Indian Name: *Punarnava*

Origin, Distribution and Composition

Hog weed is a creeping and spreading perennial herb, with a stout root-stock and many erect or spreading branches. It grows upto 2 metres in length. The leaves of the plant are simple, broad, somewhat rough, thick and brittle. The flowers are pink or red in colour. The fruits are oval in shape, dull-green or brownish in colour and about the size of caraway bean.

Hog weed is indigenous to India. It grows wild all over the country as a common creeping weed and is specially abundant during the rains.

The plant contains a crystalline acid known as boerhavic acid, potassium nitrate and a brown mass consisting of tannins, phlobaphenes and reducing sugars. The active principle of hog weed is the alkaloid punarnavine. The drug contains large quantities of potassium salts, which accounts for its diuretic properties.

Healing Power and Curative Properties

The herb has been used in indigenous medicine from time immemorial. It is laxative and produces a cooling sensation. In large doses it induces vomiting. Medicinally, the most important part of the herb is the root. It has a bitter and nauseous taste. It is beneficial in the treatment of several common ailments.

Dropsy

Hog weed increases the secretion and discharge of urine. It is effective in the treatment of dropsy, a disease marked by an excessive collection of a watery fluid in the tissues and cavities or natural hollows of the body. The fresh boiled herb should be given in the treatment of this disease. A liquid extract of the fresh or dry plant can also be given in doses of 4 to 16 grams.

Ascities

The herb is useful in the treatment of ascites, a disease characterised by accumulation of fluid inside the peritoneal cavity of the abdomen. Much more powerful effect on certain types of ascites—that is, those caused due to the cirrhosis of the liver and chronic peritonitis—than some of the other important diuretics known. The herb can be administered in the same manner as for dropsy.

Stomach Disorders

The drug is useful in strengthening the stomach and promoting its action. It is beneficial in the treatment of several stomach disorders, particularly intestinal colic. A powder of the root is given in doses of 5 grams thrice a day. It is also useful in killing or expelling intestinal worms.

Asthma

Hog weed promotes the removal of catarrhal matter and phlegm from the bronchial tubes. It is, therefore, beneficial in the treatment of asthma. A powder of the root can be taken in small doses three times a day.

Fevers

Hog weed is beneficial in the treatment of fevers. It brings down temperature by inducing copious perspiration.

Other Diseases

The root of the plant is useful in the treatment of several diseases—particularly of the kidney and heart—as well as gonorrhoea. It is also valuable in oedema, anaemia, cough, pluerisy, nervous weakness, constipation and paralysis.

Skin Diseases

The root of the plant is an effective remedy for several skin diseases. A paste of the root can be applied beneficially as a dressing for oedematous swellings. A hot poultice of the root can be applied with gratifying results to ulcers, abscesses and similar skin diseases. It is also used for extracting guinea-worms. Charaka, the great physician of ancient India, used it in the form of ointment in leprosy and other skin diseases.

Holy Basil

Botanical Name: *Ocimum sanctum*
Indian Name: *Tulsi*

Origin, Distribution and Composition

Holy basil is a many branched, erect, stout and aromatic herb. It grows upto the height of about 75 cms and is hairy all over. The plant has tender, egg-shaped leaves, usually smooth, upto 2.5 cm in length, small, purplish or reddish flowers in small compact clusters on slender spikes, small fruits and yellowish or reddish seeds. The herb is bitter and pungent.

It is grown in flower pots in most Hindu homes. Its leaves are used in the worship of gods and goddesses and partaken as *prasad*.

This herb has been known from as early as the vedic period. Hindus regard it as an earthly manifestation of goddess Vrindavani who is dear to Lord Vishnu.

The holy basil is native to India. It reached Western Europe only in the 16th century. It has now been widely grown throughout the world.

The leaves of holy basil yield an essential oil which contains eugenol, carvacrol, methyl eugenol and caryophyllene. It has the property of destroying bacteria and insects. The leaves have also been separated to yield ursolic acid, apigenin, luteolin, apigenin-7, glucuronid, orientin and molludistin.

Healing Power and Curative Properties

The plant has medicinal properties. The leaves are nerve tonic and sharpen memory. They promote the removal of catarrhal matter and phlegm from the bronchial tubes. The leaves strengthen the stomach and induce copious perspiration. The seeds of the plant are mucilaginous or starchy and nourishing. They have a soothing effect on the skin and the mucous membranes. They also increase the volume of urine.

Fevers

The leaves of basil are specific for many fevers. During the rainy season, when malaria and dengue fever are widely prevalent, tender leaves, boiled with tea, act as a preventive against these diseases. In case of acute fevers, a decoction of the leaves boiled with powdered cardamom in half a litre of water and mixed with sugar and milk brings down the temperature.

Sore Throat

Water boiled with basil leaves can be taken as a drink in case of sore throat. This water can also be used as a gargle.

Respiratory Disorders

The herb is useful in the treatment of respiratory system disorders. A decoction of the leaves, with honey and ginger is an effective remedy for bronchitis, asthma, influenza, cough and cold. A decoction of the leaves, cloves and common salt also gives immediate relief in case of influenza. They should be boiled in half a litre of water till only half the water is left and then taken.

Kidney Stones

Basil has strengthening effect on the kidney. In case of renal stones, the juice of basil leaves and honey, if taken regularly for six months, will expel them via the urinary tract.

Heart Disorders

Basil has a beneficial effect in cardiac disease and the weakness resulting from them. It reduces the level of blood cholesterol.

Children's Ailments

Common paediatric problems like cough, cold, fever, diarrhoea and vomiting respond favourably to the juice of basil leaves. If pustules of chicken pox delay their appearance, basil leaves taken with saffron will hasten them.

Stress

Basil leaves are regarded as an adaptogen or anti-stress agent. Recent studies have shown that the leaves afford significant protection against stress. Even healthy persons can chew 12 leaves of basil, twice a day, to prevent stress. It purifies blood and helps prevent several common ailments.

Mouth Infections

The leaves are quite effective for the ulcers and infections in the mouth. A few leaves chewed will cure these condtions.

Insect Bites

The herb is a prophylactic or preventive and curative for insect stings or bites. A teaspoon of the juice of the leaves is taken and repeated after a few hours. Fresh juice must also be applied to the affected parts. A paste of the fresh roots is also effective in cases of bites of insects and leeches.

Skin Disorders

Applied locally, basil juice is beneficial in the treatment of ringworm and other skin diseases. It has also been tried successfully by some naturopaths in the treatment of leucoderma.

Eye Disorders

Basil juice is an effective remedy for sore eyes and night-blindness, which is generally caused by deficiency of vitamin A. Two drops of black basil juice should be put into the eyes daily at bedtime.

Teeth Disorders

The herb is useful in teeth disorders. Its leaves, dried in the sun and powdered, can be used for brushing teeth. It can also be mixed with mustard oil to make a paste and used as tooth paste. This is very good for maintaining dental health, counteracting bad breath and for massaging the gums. It is also useful in pyorrhoea and other teeth disorders.

Headaches

Basil makes a good medicine for headache. A decoction of the leaves can be given for this disorder. Pounded leaves mixed with sandalwood paste can also be applied on the forehead for getting relief from heat, headache and for providing coolness in general.

Other Diseases

A decoction of the leaves can be given with beneficial results in gout and gonorrhoea. This decoction is also useful in neuralgia. The juice of the leaves is a well-known remedy for earache and dullness of hearing. A few drops of the juice can be put in the ear for the treatment of these conditions. The powder of the leaves is used as snuff for expelling maggots from the nose.

The seeds of the plant are useful in diarrhoea, chronic dysentery, habitual constipation, gonorrhoea, internal piles, cough, kidney disorders and fever. The mucilaginous jelly, formed by infusing 4 to 12 grams of the seeds in cold water for sometime, can be taken with sugar to treat these diseases. The cold infusion can also be taken for relieving pain after childbirth. A poultice of the seeds are beneficial for sores and sinuses.

Indian Gooseberry

Botanical Name: *Emblica officinalis*
Indian Name: *Amla*

Origin, Distribution and Composition

Indian gooseberry is a small or middle-sized deciduous tree. It has small, very closely set, 10 to 13 mm long, leaves. The branches of the tree appear feathery. The tree has pale green flowers usually in small dense clusters below the leaves. The fruits are fleshy, round with its contour indistinctly marked into 6 lobes, about 1.5 to 2.5 cms in diameter and, pale green or yellowish in colour. The fruit has a seed inside with three angles and three sides.

Indian gooseberry has been used as a valuable ingredient of various medicines in India and the Middle East from time immemorial. Shusrut, the great authority on *Ayurveda*, considers it the best of all acid fruits and most useful for health and in treating diseases. It is said that the ancient sage *Muni* Chyawan rejuvenated himself in his late 70's and regained virility with its use.

As the name suggests the Indian gooseberry is indigenous to India. An analysis shows that it contains on an average, moisture 81.8 per cent, protein 0.5 per cent, fat 0.1 per cent, minerals 0.5 per cent, fibre 3.4 per cent and carbohydrates 13.7 per cent, per 100 grams of edible portion. Its mineral and vitamin contents include calcium, phosphorus, iron, carotene, thiamine, riboflavin, niacin and vitamin C. Its calorific value is 58.

It is valued chiefly for its high vitamin C content. Repeated laboratory tests show that every 100 grams of fresh fruit provides 470 to 680 mgs of vitamin C. The vitamin C value of *amla* increases further when the juice is extracted from the fruit. The dehydrated berry provides 2428 to 3470 mgs of vimtain C per 100 grams. Even when it is dried in shade and turned into powder, it retains as much as 1780 to 2660 mgs of vitamin C.

The seeds of the Indian gooseberry contain a fixed oil, phosphatides and an essential oil. The fruits, bark and the leaves of the tree are rich in tannin.

Healing Power and Curative Properties

Indian gooseberry is a wonder herb and one of the precious gifts of nature to man. It contributes greatly towards health and longevity. Ayurvedic physicians and *hakims* use this herb very commonly in their medicines and regard it as a medicine for heart and other health problems. They also advise its external application due to its cool and astringent properties.

The fruit is acrid, cooling, refreshing and laxative. It increases the volume of urine. The raw fruit is a mild purgative. The flowers of the tree are cooling, refreshing and mild purgative. The root and bark of the tree are useful in arresting secretion or bleeding. A tablespoon each of fresh gooseberry juice and honey mixed together is a very valuable medicine for the treatment of several ailments. Its regular use every morning promotes vigour in the body within a few days. When fresh fruit is not available, dry powder can be mixed with honey.

Respiratory Disorders

Indian gooseberry is beneficial in the treatment of respiratory disorders. It is especially valuable in tuberculosis of the lungs, asthma and bronchitis.

Diabetes

This herb, due to its high vitamin C content, is effective in controling diabetes. A tablespoon of its juice, mixed with a cup of fresh bitter-gourd juice, taken daily for two months will stimulate the pancreas and enable it to secrete insulin, thus reducing the blood sugar in diabetes. Diet restrictions should be strictly observed while taking this medicine. It will also prevent eye complications in diabetes.

Equal quantities of powdered *amla*, jambul fruit and bitter-gourd provide a very useful remedy for diabetes. A tablespoon of this mixture once or twice a day would be effective in checking the progress of the disease.

Heart Disorders

Indian gooseberry is considered an effective remedy for heart disease. It tones up the functions of all the organs of the body and builds up health by destroying the heterogenous or harmful and disease causing elements. It also renewes energy.

Eye Disorders

The juice of Indian gooseberry with honey is useful in preserving eye sight. It is beneficial in the treatment of conjuctivitis and glaucoma. It reduces intraocular tension in a remarkable manner. A cup of this juice mixed with honey can be taken twice daily for this condition.

Rheumatism

To treat rheumatism, a teaspoon of the powder of the dry fruit mixed with 2 teaspoons of jaggery can be taken twice daily for a month.

Scurvy

As an extremely rich source of vitamin C, Indian gooseberry is one of the best remedies for scurvy. Powder of the dry herb, mixed with an equal quantity of sugar, can be taken in doses of 1 teaspoon, thrice daily with milk.

Diarrhoea and Dysentery

The dried fruit is also useful in diarrhoea and dysentery. A drink made from *amla,* mixed with lemon juice and *misri*---that is, sugar candy---controls acute bacillary dysentery. One tablespoon of the paste of leaves, mixed with honey or buttermilk, can be taken for treating the condition.

Ageing

Indian gooseberry has revitalising effects, as it contains an element which is very valuable in preventing ageing and in maintaining strength in old age. It improves body resistance and protects the body against infection. It strengthens the heart, hair and different glands in the body.

Other Uses

Hair Tonic: Indian gooseberry is an accepted hair tonic in traditional recipes for enriching hair growth and pigmentation. The fruit, cut into pieces, is dried, preferably in the shade. These pieces are boiled in coconut oil till the solid matter becomes charred. This darkish oil is excellent in preventing greying. The water in which dried amla pieces are soaked overnight is also nourishing to hair and can be used for the last rinse while washing the hair.

Indian gooseberry is used in various ways. The best way to take it with the least loss of vitmain C, is to eat it raw with a little salt. It is often used in the form of pickles and marmalade. It can be preserved for a long period when it is dried and powdered. The berry may also be used as a vegetable. It is boiled in a small amount of water till soft and taken with a little salt.

Indian Hemp

Botanical Name: *Cannabis sativa*
Indian Name: *Bhang or Ganja*

Origin, Distribution and Composition

Indian Hemp is a robust, tall, erect, annual herb, 1 to 5 metres high, usually with male and female plants in roughly equal numbers. It has angular stems bearing palmately or hand shaped divided leaves with greenish flowers. The hemp plant provides three products, namely, fibre from the stems, oil from the seeds and narcotic from the leaves and flowers.

The hemp plant was originally a native of Western and Central Asia. It has been cultivated since ancient times in Asia and Europe. The plant is said to have reached China more than 4,500 years ago. It spread to the New World in post-Columbian times.

In India cultivation of this plant is controlled and permitted only in the districts of Almora, Garhwal and Nainital (excluding the Terai and Bhabar) in U.P. To a small extent it is also cultivated in Kashmir, Travancore and Nepal.

The chief constituents of Indian hemp are cannabinol, pseudocannabinol and cannabinin. It also contains cannin, a resin. The biological activity of cannabis is due to alcoholic and phenolic compounds. The resin contains a crystalline compound, cannin.

Healing Power and Curative Properties

Preparations of Indian hemp have been in use as intoxicants in Asiatic countries and Africa from time immemorial. *Bhang, ganja* and *charas* have been habitually used in these parts of the world. Its narcotic and anodyne properties were appreciated by Western medical men in the early years of the last century and was incorporated in the British and United States pharmacopoeias.

The leaves of the plant are used as a drug to reduce excitement, irritation and pain as well as to induce deep sleep. They are also used as a drug to counteract spasmodic disorders, to increase the secretion and discharge of urine and arrest any secretion or bleeding. As a sedative and anodyne, they are given in doses of 2.5 grams.

Three types of narcotics are produced from the hemp plant, namely *bhang* or *hashish* which constitute the dried leaves and flowering shoots of male and female plants---has a low resin content. *Ganja* which is the dried unfertilized female inflorescences of special varieties grown in India and *charas*, which is the crude resin collected by rubbing the tops of the plant with the hands or beating them with a cloth. In all these drugs, the active principle is a resin from the glandular hairs on its leaves, stems and inflorescences.

Diarrhoea and Dysentery

The leaves are beneficial in the treatment of diarrhoea and dysentery. Two grams of dried leaves can be taken with sugar and black pepper.

Insomnia

The leaves help in insomnia. They can be administered to induce sleep where opium cannot be used. *Charas* which is the active principle of hemp, as well as *ganja,* are effective drugs to induce deep sleep.

Digestive Disorders

Bhang or *hashish* is considered useful in digestive disorders like dyspepsia and other bowel complaints. It also acts as an appetizer when taken in small doses.

Nervous Disorders

Charas is of great value in periodical headaches, migraine, acute mania, insanity and delirium, nervous vomiting, nervous exhaustion, convulsions and neuralgia. It should be taken in 1.5 to 6 centigram doses.

Gonorrhoea

The seeds of the plant are not narcotic. Their infusion is useful in gonorrhoea. *Bhang* or *hashish* can also be taken in this disorder.

Dandruff

The juice of Indian hemp removes dandruff and head lice.

Skin Disorders

A paste of the fresh leaves is useful in resolving tumours.[1] The powder of the leaves serves as a useful dressing for wounds and sores. *Ganja* is externally applied to relieve pain in itchy skin diseases.

Precautions: Excessive consumption of hemp is physically and mentally harmful. If consumed for long time, it causes loss of appetite and gastric derangment. Hemp drugs act chiefly on the cerebrum wherein they resemble the action of alcohol or opium.

Other Uses

Poisoning: The smoke from burning *ganja* is inhaled as an antidote to poisoning by orpiment, an arsenic mineral used as yellow dye and artist's pigment.

As a narcotic, hemp is consumed by itself or as a beverage. It is more often used for smoking for euphorbic purposes. Excessive smoking is harmful and may cause insanity. Hemp seed is used for the production of a drying oil and the fibre is used in making ropes.

Indian Pennywort

Botanical Name: *Centella asiatica*
Indian Name: *Khulakudi or Brahmamanduki*

Origin, Distribution and Composition

Indian pennywort is a perennial wild creeper which grows horizontally and is small and smooth. It has slender branches and small internodes. A number of leaves shoot out at each node on the upper side and numerous roots grow into the soil at each node. The creeper thus has abundant leaf growth and new plants

---

1. J.F. Dastur, *Medicinal Plants of India and Pakistan*, p. 44, D.B. Taraporevala Sons & Co. Pvt. Ltd., Bombay, 1985.

shoot out of various nodes.

The leaves of the plant are simple or of one blade, thickish, almost round or kidney-shaped and yellowish green in colour. The fruits are small, flat circular and hard. The fresh leaves have an aroma due to the presence of an oily matter called vellarine. The aroma is lost on drying

Indian pennywort is indigenous to India. It was known to Sanskrit writers from ancient times. This plant is found throughout India both in the plains and hilly tracts upto 2000 metres. It grows abundantly in moist areas and river banks, thriving in shade.

Several other substances have been isolated from the herb. These include an essential oil, a fatty oil, sitosterol, tannin and a resinous substance. The dry plant yields an alkaloid, hydrocotylin. The leaves and roots contain a bitter principle, vellarine, pectic acid and resin. The leaves of the plant have a mixed taste—sweet, sour, astringent and bitter. The cellulose content is very low.

Healing Power and Curative Properties

The herb corrects the disordered processes of nutrition, by which organism ingests, digests, absorbs, utilizes and excretes food substances---and restores the normal function of the system. It counteracts inflammation and is a mild purgative. It also increases the secretion and discharge of urine.

All the parts of the creeper are used both for therapeutic and culinary purposes.

Improving Memory

The leaves of the Indian pennywort are considered beneficial in improving memory. The powder of the leaves taken with milk in small doses for this purpose helps in correcting the disorders.

Dysentery in Children

The leaves of the plant are an effective remedy in the early stages of dysentery in children. Three or four leaves can be taken with cumin and sugar in addition to applying a paste of the leaves on the navel.

Bowel Complaints

In case of bowel complaints amongst children, half a cup of

an infusion of its leaves with fenugreek (*methi*) can be taken, in a single dose.

Nervous Disorders

The herb is effective in nervous disorders including nervous debility. A powder of the leaves dried in shade and taken in doses of 3 to 6 decigrams, thrice a day for adults, is effective. Reduce the dose to 0.75 to 2.5 decigrams for children.

Female Sterility

Indian pennywort is effective in female sterility when combined with another herb called *chotakulpha*, (*trichodesma Indicum*). The two herbs should be uprooted when matured and dried in the shade for use. An equal quantity of both herbs should be taken, powdered with sugar candy in the ratio 2:1. Three grams of this powder should be taken both in the morning and evening with cow's milk for 3 consecutive days after menstruation. However, the woman using this recipe should be free from menstrual pain, leucorrhoea, obesity or any such disease. If she has any, these should be treated before going in for this remedy.

Elephantiasis

The drug is useful in treating elephantiasis of the scrotum and legs, which is marked by gross swelling. The juice extracted from a portion of the fresh plant or the dried stem and leaves of the plant ground with water, should be applied locally to the affected parts. A poultice of the fresh leaves or an ointment made of four grams of the leaf extract with 30 grams of lanoline is equally efficacious.

Skin Disorders

Indian pennywort is a common household remedy for skin diseases like chronic and persistent eczema, chronic ulcers and syphilitic sores. A fine powder of the dried leaves can be used as a dust in skin eruptions and syphilic ulcers. To check fever associated with these diseases, the juice of the leaves should be taken thrice a day in doses of 1 to 5 drops.

Dosage: The drug is generally given as a decoction in doses of 30 to 60 ml or as powder in doses of 2 to 6 decigrams thrice a day. The leaves of the plant can be taken in doses of 30 to 60 grams. The juice of the leaves can be taken in doses of 60 to 100 ml and the decoction of the leaves from 120 to 150 ml.

Precautions: It is advisable to take the raw juice of the leaf in small doses as the juice is very potent and an excess intake may lead to coma.

Other Uses

The leaves of Indian pennywort have culinary uses too and can be used for making soup, raw chutney, tea, raw juice and chapatis (mixed with wheat flour).

Indian Sorrel

Botanical Name: *Oxalis corniculata*
Indian Name: *Amboti-ki-patti*

Origin, Distribution and Composition

Indian sorrel is a small, hairy, annual herb. It has numerous branches which shoot out from the roots and creep to a length of 12 to 30 cms. The stem of the plant is very thin, delicate and hairy. It has pale green compound leaves, with delicate, very thin and smooth leaflets. It also has yellow flowers and cylindrical fruits containing many tiny seeds.

The herb is indigenous to India. Thriving in moisture, it grows wild during monsoon and on wet grounds. The flowers of the plant are sour due to a high content of oxalic acid and potassium oxalate.The herb is rich in vitamin B_1, iron and calcium. The leaves contain a small amount of cellulose.

Healing Power and Curative Properties

The leaves are acrid, bitter and mildly astringent. It has a predominently acid taste. It is advisable to mix the herb with other milder tasting herbs. The juice of 15 grams of this herb, mixed with five grams of basil (*tulsi*) juice, may be taken with 100 ml of tender coconut water. This raw juice can also be mixed with cooked greens. The leaves have a cooling effect and act as an appetizer.

Fevers

The leaves are useful in relieving symptoms of fever. An infusion of the leaves can bring temperature down.

Scurvy

The leaves are antiscorbutic and are useful in the prevention and treatment of scurvy—a deficiency caused by lack of vitamin C. An infusion of the leaves can be taken for this purpose.

Stomach Disorders

Fresh leaves of the plant are useful in stimulating the stomach and aiding its action. The leaves can also be eaten as an appetizer.

The leaves are beneficial in mild cases of dysentery and enteritis. They should be boiled in butter-milk and given twice a day. Fresh juice of the leaves, mixed with honey or sugar, is also useful in dysentery.

Jaundice

The herb is beneficial in the treatment of jaundice. A tablespoon of fresh juice mixed with butter-milk made of cow's milk can be taken once daily in the treatment of this disease.

Excessive Thirst

Indian sorrel curbs excessive thirst caused by diabetes or severe heat. The same method of intake as for jaundice can be followed.

Skin Disorders

The leaves are useful in certain skin diseases like warts, corns and other excrescences of the skin. They can be locally applied in these conditions. The juice of the whole plant mixed with onion is also applied to remove warts. A poultice of the leaves applied over an inflammation relieves pain, and when applied over boils, ripens them. The juice mixed with black pepper and *ghee*, gives relief from red spots and eruptions on the skin caused by biliousness.

Eye Disorders

The herb is very useful in the prevention and treatment of eye disorders. A few drops of the leaf juice put into the eyes every day keeps the eyes free from strain and prevents opacity of the cornea and cataract. The leaves are quite effective when applied locally for correcting the opacity of cornea.

Insomnia

The juice of the leaves mixed with castor oil is useful in insomnia. The juice should be mixed in an equal quantity of castor oil and heated to remove the watery content. It should then be cooled and stored in a bottle. When the scalp is massaged with this oil before going to bed, it will induce good sleep and also provide coolness to the eyes.

Precautions: As the Indian sorrel contains high concentration of oxalic acid, its use should be avoided by persons suffering from gout, rheumatism and calculi or stone in the urinary tract.

Indian Spikenard

Botanical Name: *Nardostachys jatamansi*
Indian Name: *Jatamansi*

Origin, Distribution and Composition

Indian spikenard, also known as Indian vallerine, is a perennial herb which grows upto 60 cms. It has long, woody rhizomes or an underground stem producing roots covered with fibres and small bunches of pale, pink or blue flowers. The dried rhizomes and roots of this plant constitute the drug. The Indian name *jatamansi* refers to the bearded appearance of rhizomes.

This drug is one of the first 12 drugs mentioned in the earliest European medical work, *Pharmacoepea of Hippocrates,* and has been in use in India for over 3,000 years. It is an excellent substitute for the drug, Velerian, botanically known as *Valeriana.*

The plant occurs on alpine Himalayas especially at higher attitudes of 3,000 and 4,500 metres, extending eastward from Kumaon to Sikkim and Bhutan.

The Indian spikenard yields a volatile oil, which contains an unidentified ester, an alcohol and two alkaloids. The rhizomes of the plant contain *jatamansi* acid, and an essential oil, which has the same uses as the rhizome. As an aromatic, it is an ingredient of many medicinal preparations.

Healing Power and Curative Properties

The root of the plant is aromatic, stimulant, bitter tonic and antiseptic. It is useful in counteracting spasmodic disorders, and facilitates secretion or excretion by the natural passages or pores of the body, including urine.

Nervous and Convulsive Disorders

Jatamansi can be used in the treatment of several nervous and convulsive disorders such as hysteria, epileptic fits, and certain disturbances caused by menopause. In very small doses it soothes the nervous system and acts as a tranquiliser.

Intestinal Worms

The drug is useful in treating intestinal worms. It can be given to children with a purgative like jalap. For the treatment of threadworms, an enema made of an infusion of the rhizomes can be given.

Respiratory Disorders

Jatamansi can be used in the treatment of bronchitis and other disorders of the respiratory system. Doses of 30 to 40 grains with the addition of a little camphor and cinnamon can be taken. It can also be taken as an infusion in doses of 30 to 60 grams, thrice a day.

Menstrual Disorders

The herb aids menstruation and regulates the menstrual cycle. It is specially useful in dysmenorrhoea—that is, painful and difficult menstruation.

Palpitation of the Heart

It is a good cardiac stimulant, and hence useful in treating palpitation of the heart.

Low Blood Pressure

Research has established that it helps in the treatment of low blood pressure, nervousness and intermittent pulse.

Other Uses

Hair Tonic: *Jatamansi* is a well-known hair tonic. It is an important ingredient of many hair washes and hair oils.

Ispaghula

Botanical Name: *Plantago ovata*
Indian Name: *Ishabgul*

Origin, Distribution and Composition

Ispaghula, also known as spogel seeds, is an almost stemless small herb covered with dense and soft hairy growth. It has very narrow leaves and minute flowers in oval or cylindrical spikes. The upper half of its fruits opens like a lid and its seeds are boat shaped. The seeds of this plant, also known as fleaseeds, constitute the drug.

Ispaghula is indigenous to India, and has been used extensively in the Indian system of medicine from ancient times. It was prescribed by ancient physicians as a cure for inflammatory and functional derangements of the mucous membranes of the gastro-intestinal and genito-urinary system.

The seeds contain a large amount of mucilage and a small amount of holoside planteose. The seeds also show the presence of a number of amino acids in the combined form, namely valine, alanine, glycine, glutamic acid, cystine, lysine, leucine and tyrosine. Valine, alanine and glutamic acid are also found in their free form. The Ispaghula embryo oil has been reported to be a good source of linoleic acid.

Healing Power and Curative Properties

The medicinal properties of the seeds are largely due to the large amount of mucilage and albuminous matter present in them. The seeds are cooling and mildly laxative. They act as a diuretic and also have a soothing effect on the skin and mucous membranes.

Ispaghula husk *(Ishabgul-ki-bhusi)* is the dry seed-cover of the plant, obtained by crushing the seeds and separating the husk by winnowing. The husk has similar properties as the seeds. It has also the advantage of passing smoothly through alimentary canal without causing irritation. The husk can be taken dry and is easier to use than the whole seeds.

Constipation

Due to its soothing effect on the mucous membranes Ispaghula is used in constipation. The seeds should be soaked in water before use, which makes them disintegrate in the alimentary canal. The large amount of mucilage in the seeds binds and increases the mass of the stool, thus smoothening its passage. The action is, chiefly mechanical, rather than physiological. Two tablespoons of the seeds should be taken with milk or water in this condition. The seeds are particularly useful in chronic constipation characterised by spasms.

Dysentery

Ispaghula seeds are a popular remedy for several kinds of chronic dysentery and diarrhoea. In case of heaviness in the stomach and the intestines in dysentery, about 50 grams of castor oil should be administered with milk to ease out hard lumps of stools. When a few motions have cleared the intestines, 12 grams of ispaghula seeds mixed with about 100 grams of curd should be taken three to four times in the day.

A mixture of 180 grams each of the seeds and sugar candy given three or four times a day is an effective remedy for slimy dysentery. For chronic diarrhoea and dysentery, the seeds can be taken either as a decoction or infusion of powder with sugar.

Abdominal Pain

Ispaghula is useful in treating frequent griping in the belly caused by stomach ulcers. The seeds with husk are soaked in water or milk for a few hours. The liquid is strained and can be taken at night. The high mucilaginous content in the herb forms a covering inside the intestinal wall which protects the lining mucosa and helps in the healing of ulcers. Irritation and gripe will also decrease.

Piles

Ispaghula seeds are one of the most effective remedies for piles. While the high mucilage content in this herb cures constipation, the rich tannin content cures inflammation and ulceration in the intestinal tract up to the anus. This double action helps cure piles.

Arteriosclerosis

The embryo oil of the seeds, having 50 per cent linoleic acid, prevents arteriosclerosis. This oil is more active than safflower oil, and has been found to reduce the serum cholesterol level in rabbits.

Gonorrhoea

Ispaghula is very useful in the treatment of gonorrhoea because of its diuretic and soothing properties.

Whitlow

Ispaghula is an effective remedy in whitlow affecting the pulp of the fingertip with an abcess. About 12 grams of ispaghula should be soaked in 45 grams of vinegar and applied to the spot when the whole thing has swollen. The poultice-like mixture should be bandaged with a clean cloth and water sprinkled over it. The bandage should be changed every 3 hours. The inflammation will subside within 3 days.

Rheumatism

An emollient poultice made of the seeds with vinegar and oil is useful for rheumatism and gout.

Kantakari

Botanical Name: *Solanum xanthocarpum*
Indian Name: *Kateli*

Origin, Distribution and Composition

Kantakari, also known as Indian Solanum, is a prickly, branches-perennial herb. The branches are densely covered with minute star-shaped hairs. The plant has yellow, shining prickles of about 1.5 cm in size. it has very prickly, sparsely hairy, egg-shaped leaves; purple flowers, round fruits, yellow in colour with green veins and numerous smooth seeds. The fruit of the plant constitutes the drug.

Kantakari is indigenous to India. The plant occurs throughout India, often in waste lands, on roadsides and in open scrublands.

The fruit of the plant yields carpesteral, glucoside-alkaloids and solanocarpine. It also yields glucoside-alkaloids, solamine-S. On hydrolysis it yields alkaloid solanidine-S.

Healing Power and Curative Properties

The root is one of the important medicinal ingredients used by the physicians of Ayurveda, who use it to treat several common ailments. The drug is bitter in taste and a mild purgative. Experiments have shown that the fruits and shoots of the plant possess antibacterial properties.

Respiratory Disorders

Kantakari is useful in clearing catarrh and phelgm from the bronchial tubes. It is therefore used in the treatment of respiratory diseases like asthma, bronchitis and cough.

Stomach Disorders

The herb can be used to treat constipation and flatulence. It strengthens the stomach and promotes its action. It corrects disordered processes of nutrition by which the organism ingests, digests, absorbs, utilises and excretes food substances and restores normal function of the system. The drug also possesses anthelminitic (worm destroying) property and is useful in eliminating intestinal worms.

Dropsy

Kantakari is useful in the treatment of dropsy, a disease marked by an excessive collection of a fluids in the tissues and cavities or natural hollows of the body. The drug helps increase the secretion and discharge of urine.

Throat Disorders

The herb is especially useful in throat disorders like sore throat and tonsilitis. An extract of the plant should be used as a gargle in such cases. This is prepared by continuously boiling the plant in about 2 litres of water after washing it thoroughly, till it reduces to half its volume and it should be filtered.

Gum Diseases

The extract of the plant, prepared as for throat disorders, is also very useful in gum diseases. For better results, black mustard should be boiled along with the plant.

Snake Bites

The root of the plant has been traditionally used in snake and scorpion bites. A paste of the root can be prepared by grinding it on a stone with lemon juice and applying to the affected part. The patient should be taken to the doctor immediately.

Other Diseases

The drug is also useful in treating several other diseases like heart disease, chest pain, certain types of fever, muscular pains, gonorrhoea, dysuria, enlargement of the liver and spleen and stone in the urinary bladder. The fruit of the plant is also considered useful in treating sore throat, bronchitis, muscular pains and fevers.

Dosages: The herb can be used either in the form of confection, decoction or juice. The decoction is taken in doses of 15 ml to 60 ml. The juice is taken in doses ranging from 2 ml to 8 ml.

Other Uses

Tender leaves and fruits are eaten as a vegetable after cooking.

Liquorice

Botanical Name: *Glycyrrhiza glabra*
Indian Name: *Mulethi*

Origin, Distribution and Composition

Liquorice is a popular flavouring agent. It is a tall, erect herb, growing upto about 1.5 metres in height. It has compound leaves, lilac or light violet flowers, flat fruit and is densely covered with small spinous outgrowths. The dried roots and underground stems or rhizomes of the plant constitute the drug.

Liquorice has been known to pharmacists for thousands of years. In ancient Chinese pharmacy, it was used for its rejuvenating properties especially when used for long periods. It was used to quench thirst, alleviate feverishness, pain, cough and distress of breathing.

Liquorice plays an important part in Ayurvedic system of medicine and is one of the principal drugs mentioned by Susruta.

Liquorice is cultivated in southern Europe, Syria, Iraq, Turkey, Greece and Russia. Large quantities of these roots are annually imported in India, though it is also cultivated in north-west parts of the country.

The herb contains glycyrrhizin, glycyrrhizic acid and glycyrrhetinic acid.

Healing Power and Curative Properties

The root of the plant is a laxative and expectorant. When externally used it has a soothing effect on the skin. Powdered liquorice is very popular in allopathic medicine.

Stomach Disorders

Liquorice is an excellent remedy for relieving pain, discomfort and other symptoms caused by acrid matter in the stomach. It should be taken in powder form.

Sore Throat

The herb is a recognized home remedy for sore throat. A small piece of raw liquorice if chewed or sucked, provides relief by soothing the inflammation.

Cough

Lubricating the throat with a decoction of liquorice mixed with honey brings relief in dry cough.

Myopia

Liquorice is used in the treatment of myopia. Half a teaspoon of the powder of the root, mixed with an equal amount of honey and half the quantity of *ghee*, can be given twice daily with milk on an empty stomach in this case.

Constipation

Liquorice is also used as a laxative in constipation. Its Powder is taken with jaggery and water in this condition.

Stomach Ulcer

Liquorice is very effective in treating pain due to stomach ulcers, as it soothes the irritation caused by acids. Pieces of the dried root soaked overnight in water and the infusion taken with rice gruel helps in the cure of ulcers. Even allopathic physicians use liquorice for treating ulcers.

Muscular Pains

Liquorice alleviates muscular pains. Taking an infusion of the roots soaked overnight relieves any chronic joint problems.

Mouth Disorders

The sticks of dried rhizomes are soaked in water and the infusion used as a gargle brings quick relief in oral inflammations. Tiny bits of the stick with sugar-candy can also be sucked.

Baldness

The herb is effective in treating patchy baldness. Small pieces of the root are ground in milk with a pinch of saffron to a paste. When this paste is applied over the bald patches at bedtime regularly, hair growth is seen within a few weeks. This prescription is very effective in the initial stages of baldness, excessive hair loss and dandruff.

Wounds and Scalds

Liquorice powder mixed with butter or *ghee* and honey, can be applied on cuts and wounds with good results. The leaves of the plant, applied as a poultice, is a useful remedy in scalds of the head and body.

Corns

The herb heals corns which are just appearing. A paste of liquorice sticks mixed with sesame or mustard oil,if rubbed into the hardened skin at bed time softens the skin and the corn decreases in size.

Precautions: Continuous and uninterrupted use of liquorice in the treatment of stomach ulcer is not advisable as it may cause increase in weight and puffiness of body. It should also be avoided in pregnancy and in heart and kidney conditions.

Madhuca

Botanical Name: *Madhuca indica*
Indian Name: *Mahua*

Origin, Distribution and Composition

Madhuca, also known as butter tree, is a large deciduous tree, 20 metres in height with a spreading top. It has thick leathery leaves and small, fleshy, pale or dull white musk-scented flowers in clusters near the end of branches. Its fruits are fleshy, greenish, with brown and shining seeds.

The bark, leaves, flowers and seeds of the tree constitute the drug. The trade name, madhuca, is based on the Sanskrit name of the plant.

The tree is indigenous to the Central India. It is common in sub-mountainous regions of the Himalayas, and is, at certain

125

places, a chief constituent of the forest vegetation.

The leaves of the tree contain alkaloid glucosidic saponin. The seeds contain a fatty oil. Recently a new sapogenin and basic acid have also been isolated from the seeds.

Healing Power and Curative Properties

Madhuca is useful in arresting secretions or bleeding because of its tannin content. The bark of the tree is an astringent and tonic. The flowers promote the removal of catarrhal matter and phlegm from the bronchial tubes. They also exercise a soothing effect on the skin and mucous membranes. A spirit prepared from the flowers is considered to be nutritive and a tonic.

Bronchitis

The flowers of the tree are effective in bronchitis and coughs. They should be given in doses of 30 grams with 250 ml of milk.

Rheumatism

A decoction of the bark can be given internally in rheumatic diseases. The oil extracted from the seeds can also be applied locally on the affected area.

Diabetes

A decoction of the bark can also be taken in diabetes mellitus with beneficial results.

Piles

Madhuca oil extracted from the seeds has laxative properties. It helps cure piles by relieving chronic constipation.

Orchitis

Vapours of boiling madhuca leaves are useful in relieving the pain of orchitis or the inflammation of testicles.

Problem of Breast Milk Secretion

Flowers of the tree are effective in increasing the flow of milk in nursing mothers. The seeds also have a similar property.

Bleeding Gums

A lotion is made by mixing 4 ml of the liquid extract of the bark of the madhuca tree with 300 ml of water is an excellent gargle for bleeding and spongy gums.

Tonsilitis

This lotion can also be used as a gargle in the treatment of acute and chronic tonsilitis and pharyngitis.

Eczema

The leaves of madhuca are effective in the treatment of eczema. The leaves, smeared with sesame oil, warmed over a fire and bandaged on the affected parts provide relief. They should be changed after every 3 to 4 hours.

Skin Disorders

The ash of the leaves, mixed with *ghee*, is often used as a dressing for burns and scalds in the indigenous sytem of medicine. For the cure of itching, a paste of the bark is applied locally. The oil extracted from the seeds can also be applied locally in skin diseases.

Other Uses

The madhuca tree is a very important source of food for the Gonds and other tribes in Central and Western India. The flowers are eaten raw or cooked. They are also used for making alcohol, vinegar, syrups and jams. Madhuca oil is largely used in the manufacture of soaps, besides cooking.

Margosa

Botanical Name: *Azadirachta indica*
Indian Name: *Neem*

Origin, Distribution and Composition

Margosa is a very common tree in India. It is a large evergreen dense tree growing some 10 to 10.5 metre tall with a girth of about 2 to 3 metres. The leaves of this tree are divided into numerous leaflets, each resembling a full-grown leaf. The tree has small, white flowers in auxillary bunches and 1.2 to 1.8 cm long green or yellow fruits with a seed in each.

The margosa tree has played a key role in Ayurvedic medicine and agriculture since time immemorial. It is indigenous to South Asia, where up to twenty million trees line the roads. The tree occurs naturally in the Deccan peninsula, but is cultivated all over India. It is also common in Indonesia, Sri Lanka, Myanmar, Pakistan, Japan and tropical regions of Australia and Africa.

The seeds contain substantial amount of essential oil, known as margosa or *neem* oil. The bitter constituents separated from this oil are nimbin, nimbinin and nimbidin. The main active constituent of these is nimbidin which contains sulphur. The blossoms yield a glucoside, nimbosterin and a highly pungent essential oil, nimbosterol nimbecetin and fatty acids. The flowers contain a bitter substance and an irritant bitter oil. The fruits contain a bitter principle, baka yanin and the trunk bark yields nimbin, nimbidin, nimbinin and an essential oil.

Healing Power and Curative Properties

Neem tree is generally considered to be an air purifier and a preventive against malarial fever and cholera. All parts of the tree possess medicinal properties. The leaves are useful in relieving flatulence, promoting the removal of catarrhal matter and phlegm from the bronchial tubes, and in increasing secretion and discharge of urine. They also act as an insecticide. The bark is a bitter tonic and a stimulant. It arrests secretions and bleeding besides counter-acting any spasmodic disorders. The root bark has the same properties as the bark of the trunk. The gum discharged by the stem is a stimulant and tonic with a soothing effect on the skin and mucous membranes.

Malaria

An infusion or a decoction of the fresh leaves is a bitter vegetable tonic and alterative, especially in chronic malarial fevers because of its action on the liver. It should be taken in doses of 15 to 60 grams.

Piles

The use of 3 grams of the inner bark of *neem* with 6 grams of jaggery every morning, is very effective in piles. To check bleeding piles, 3 or 4 *neem* fruits can be administered with water.

Leprosy

The sap of the *neem* tree has been found effective in leprosy, when taken in daily doses of 60 grams. Simultaneously the patient's body should be massaged with the sap. This regimen should be continued for 40 days. If the sap is not available, 12 grams of *neem* leaves and three decigrams of pepper can be ground in water and taken.

Skin Disorders

The leaves, applied externally, are very useful in skin diseases. They are especially beneficial in the treatment of boils, chronic ulcers, eruptions of smallpox, syphilitic sores, glandular swellings and wounds. They can be used either as a poultice, decoction or liniment.

An ointment prepared from *neem* leaves is also very effective in healing ulcers and wounds. This ointment is prepared by frying 50 grams of the leaves in 50 grams of pure *ghee* and mashing the mixture thoroughly in the same *ghee* till an ointment consistency is obtained. A paste prepared from the bark by rubbing it in water can also be applied on wounds.

Hair Disorders

If there is any hair loss or it has ceased to grow, washing with the decoction of *neem* leaves may help. This will not only stop hair from falling but also help their growth. Frequent application of *neem* oil also destroys insects in the hair.

Eye Diseases

Neem is very useful in eye diseases. Application of the juice of *neem* leaves to the eyes every night is highly effective in the treatment of night blindness. The leaves should be pounded and made into a thin paste with water. The juice should then be pressed out through a clean piece of cloth and applied to the eyes with an eye rod.

The juice obtained by rubbing a few *neem* leaves with a little water and strained through a clean piece of cloth is useful in pain in the eyes caused by conjunctivitis. It is warmed, and a few drops put into the ear opposite the ailing eye, to give relief. Eyes are cured after a few applications.

Ear Ailments

Steam fomentation with *neem* decoction provides immediate comfort in cases of earache. A handful of neem leaves should be boiled in a litre of water and the ear fomented with the steam thus produced. The juice of *neem* leaves mixed with an equal quantity of pure honey is an effective remedy for any boils in the ear. The juice is to be warmed a little and a few drops fused in the ear. Regular application for a few days will provide relief from such ailments.

In case of an insect fluxing in the ear the juice of *neem* leaves, with some common salt,is warmed and few drops injected in the ear, kill the insect. Two drops of lukewarm *neem* oil put in the ear twice a day can cure deafness.

Oral Disorders

Cleaning the teeth regularly with a *neem* twig prevents gum diseases. It firms up loose teeth, relieves toothache, evacuates the bad odour and protects the mouth from various infections.

Other Uses

Post-Parturition Disorders: Neem is very useful at the time of child-birth. Administration of the juice of *neem* leaves to the woman in labour before childbirth produces normal contraction in the uterus and prevents possible inflammation. It corrects bowel movements and checks onset of fevers, thereby facilitating the normal delivery. The use of a tepid decoction of *neem* leaves as a vaginal douche heals any wounds caused during delivery and disinfects the vaginal passage.

Neem is a powerful insecticide to kill soil nematodes and other plant parasites and is useful as a mosquito repellant. *Neem* twig is also used as a toothbrush, and its juice in toothpastes and contraceptives.

Nutmeg

Botanical Name: *Myristica fragrans*
Indian Name: *Jaiphal*

Origin, Distribution and Composition

Nutmeg is the dried kernel of the seeds of an evergreen tree. It has a strong aroma with a slightly bitter taste. The nutmeg tree is usually 9 to 12 metres high but sometimes attains a height of upto 20 metres or more.

Nutmeg tree grows in Indonesia, Malaysia, Sri Lanka and the West Indies. It appears from ancient records that nutmeg tree flourished in India at one time, but is a scarce plant species now.

Nutmeg contains an essential oil and saponin. The dry, ripe seeds of the fruit contains a volatile oil and a fixed oil. The dry leaves of the tree yield an essential oil consisting of myristicin.

Healing Power and Curative Properties

Nutmeg was used in the preparations of various medicines in ancient times. Even today it is used in several important and widely used pharmaceutical preparations. The oil extracted from the herb is used in liniments, perfumery, hair lotions and as an antispasmodic carminative.

Digestive Disorders

The powder of nutmeg, about 5 to 15 grams, mixed with apple juice or banana, is used as a specific remedy for diarrhoea caused by indigestion of food. The same quantity of nutmeg powder taken with a tablespoon of fresh *amla* juice thrice daily, is effective for indigestion, hiccups and morning sickness.

Insomnia

The powder of nutmeg, mixed with fresh *amla* juice, is also an effective medicine for insomnia, irritability and depression. Nutmeg paste mixed with honey is given to infants who cry at night for no apparent reason, to induce sleep. It should, however, not be given regularly without medical advice as it may cause serious complications and addiction in the infants.

Dehydration

The herb is useful in treating dehydration caused by vomiting and diarrhoea, particularly in cholera. An infusion prepared from half a nutmeg in half a litre of water given with tender coconut water in doses of 15 grams at a time, is an effective treatment.

Skin Disdorders

Nutmeg is used in the treatment of skin diseases like ringworm and eczema. The paste of the herb prepared by rubbing it on a stone slab in one's own early morning saliva--- before cleansing the mouth---is applied once daily as a specific remedy in the treatment of these conditions.

Rheumatism

A nutmeg coarsely powdered and fried in *til* oil, until all the particles become brown, is very useful as an external application to relieve any rheumatic pain, neuralgia and sciatica. The oil should be cooled and strained before application.

Common Cold

In case of a running nose, a paste made from this with cow's milk and 75 mg of opium should be applied to the forehead and the nose, it will provide quick relief.

Precautions: Nutmeg should be taken in very small doses; in appreciable doses it excites the motor cortex and produces epileptic convulsions and lesions in the liver. Even a teaspoon of nutmeg can produce toxic symptoms such as burning in the stomach, nausea, vomiting, restlessness and giddiness with hallucinations.

Other Uses

Sex Stimulant: Nutmeg, mixed with honey and a half-boiled egg, makes an excellent sex tonic. It prolongs the duration of the sexual act if taken an hour before intercourse.

Onion

Botanical Name: *Allium cepa*
Indian Name: *Piyaz*

Origin, Distribution and Composition

The onion is a biennial herb, usually grown as an annual. All parts of onion produce a strong odour when crushed. It has a superficial root system, a very short flattened stem at the base, which increases in diametre as it grows. Leaves are long, linear and hollow. A bulb is formed by the thickening of the leaf base when the plant reaches a critical stage. The fruit is a spherical capsule.

Onion is one of the oldest cultivated herbs. It was a popular food in ancient Egypt, where it is depicted on tombs as early as 3200 B.C. The Sanskrit word for onion is *palandu* which has been mentioned in the *Garuda Purana*. The great Indian sage, Maharishi Atreya and Lord Dhanwantri have described the use of onions in great detail.

Onion is believed to have originated in Central Asia, possibly in the Iran-Pakistan region. It has been cultivated since ancient times in the Middle East and India. Its areas of cultivation include India, Malaysia, Indonesia, Burma, the Philippines, China, Egypt, West and East Africa, tropical South and Central America and the Caribbean.

Onion has been used as a herbal remedy from time immemorial. The physicians of ancient Egypt prescribed onions in various diseases. Dioscoredes in the first century A.D. attributed many herbal remedies to them. In 1835, the onion and milk diet was advocated for dropsy. In 1912, a French physician, Dr. Dalache published a comprehensive article on onion cure.[1]

It is high in food value, moderate in protein content and rich in calcium and riboflavin. There is considerable variation in the composition between different varieties, it also varies with the stage of maturity and the length of storage. Matured onions approximately contain moisture 86.6 per cent, protein 1.2 per cent, fat 0.1 per cent, fibre 0.6 per cent, minerals 0.4 per cent and carbohydrate 11.1 per cent, per 100 grams of edible portion. The carbohydrate is principally in the form of sugars. Its mineral and vitamin contents are calcium, phosphorus, iron, carotene, thiamine, riboflavin, niacin and vitamin C. Its calorific value is 51.

Onions contain an essential oil and organic sulphides. The scales of onion contain catechol and protocatechuic acid. The odour in onion is due to organic sulphur compounds, and is produced only when the tissues are cut or injured by enzyme action on a water-soluble amino acid. Heat or freeze-drying prevents the enzyme action, so that cooking produces a different odour, flavour and pungency.

Healing Power and Curative Properties

Onions have great therapeutic value. They are stimulants and a mild counter-irritant. They have diuretic properties and promote the removal of catarrhal matter and phelgm from the bronchial tubes.

---

1. Dr. S.J. Singh, Food Remedies, 4th edition, p. 146, Nature Cure Council of Medical Research, Lucknow, 1982.

Respiratory Diseases

Onion has the property to liquify phlegm and prevent its recurrence. It has been used as a herbal remedy for centuries in colds, coughs, bronchitis and influenza. Three to four teaspoons of onion juice and honey, mixed in equal proportion can be taken daily in treatment of these conditions. It is one of the safest preventive medicines against common cold during winter.

Tuberculosis

Though it has been known for many years that onion possessed some germicidal properties, recently two Italian doctors, E. Cuboin and C. Moriandi found that the injection of its juice prevented the development of tuberculosis in animals in whom germs of tuberculosis were injected. Patients of tuberculosis have improved following adequate consumption of onions.

Anaemia

Onions are noted for their easily assimilable iron content. They are, therefore, beneficial in treating anaemia.

Heart Attack

Recent researches in the West have established onion as an effective preventive edible against heart-attack. This benefit is due to the presence of its essential oil, aliypropyl disulphide, catechol, protocatechuic acid, thiopropiono aldehyde, thiocyanate, minerals and vitamins.

Dr. N. Radhakrishnan, Principal of the Trivandrum Medical College, and Dr. K. Madhavan Kutty have established, after seven years of research, that to get rid of the disorders due to coronary disease or blood pressure, one should take 100 grams of onion per day.[1] It assists the functioning of the heart by correcting thrombosis besides reducing blood cholesterol.

Cholera

Onion is an effective remedy for cholera. About 30 grams of onion and seven black peppers can be finely pounded and given to the patient. It allays thirst, restlessness and also lessens vomiting and diarrhoea immediately. The addition of a little

---

1. Treatment by Onions for Cure and Prevention of Disease, Prakritvani, monthly magazine, p. 9, Jan. 1988 issue, Lucknow.

sugar to the recipe will increase its effectiveness.

Urinary Disorders

Onions are highly beneficial in the treatment of the disorders of the urinary system. For burning sensation while passing urine, 6 grams of onion should be boiled in 500 grams of water. When the water is reduced to half, it should be cooled, strained and given to the patient. This relieves the burning sensation. Onion grated with water on a stone slab and mixed with 60 grams of sugar, is effective in treating retention of urine; it brings about free urination within a short time.

Piles

Onions are very effective in bleeding piles. About 30 grams of onions should be finely ground on a slab with water and 60 grams of sugar added to it. Taken twice daily this brings relief within a few days.

Teeth Disorders

Latest research by Russian doctors have confirmed the bactericidal properties of onion. According to these findings, a person consuming at least one raw onion every day after thorough mastication, is protected from a host of teeth disorders. Chewing raw onion for 3 minutes is sufficient to kill all germs in the mouth. Toothache is often alleviated by placing a small piece of onion on the affected tooth or gum.

Skin Disorders

Onion is irritating to the skin and stimulates the circulation of blood in the mucous membranes. Warts sometimes disappear when rubbed with cut onions.

Ear Disorders

Cotton wool dipped in onion juice and put into the ear is a popular Russian remedy for noises in the ears. Heated juice dropped in the ear relieves earache.

Precautions: White onion is preferable to the red and yellow varieties. Onions should be taken with meals preferably raw, as fried or cooked onions are comparatively difficult to digest. For therapeutic purposes, it is advisable to use onion juice instead of the whole onion. Its being a stimulating and irritating food, one should avoid excess consumption.

Other Uses

Aphrodisiac: Onion is one of the most important aphrodisiac foods, second only to garlic. It increases libido and strengthens the reproductive organs. The white variety of onion should be peeled off, crushed and fried in pure butter. This mixture acts as an excellent aphrodisiac tonic if taken regularly with a spoon of honey on an empty stomach.

The immature and mature bulbs are either eaten raw or cooked. They are used in soups and sauces and for seasoning many foods. Small white leaf bases—before the bulbs are formed —are eaten raw, by themselves or in salads.

Parsley

Botanical Name: *Petroselinum crispum*
Indian Name: *Prajmoda*

Origin, Distribution and Composition

Parsely is an erect, biennial or short lived perennial herb with a fleshy aromatic tap root and dark green shiny leaves which rise from a short stem. There are two groups of parsley. One group is with plain leaves and the other with curled leaves, commonly known as moss-curled.

The Romans used parsley as a remedy for sore eyes and as a tonic to increase the strength of their gladiators. The large amount of vitamin A and C contained in parsley bears out their practice.

Parsley is a native of Southern Europe. It can be grown successfully throughout the tropics, but tends to decay rather quickly near the equator. It is widely grown in the Philippines, Malaysia, East and West Africa, Brazil and the Caribbean. It is not commonly grown in India.

An analysis of parsley shows it to consist of moisture 74.6 per cent, protein 5.9 per cent, fat 1.0 per cent, minerals 3.2 per cent, fibre 1.8 per cent, carbohydrates 13.5 per cent per 100 grams of edible portion. Its mineral and vitamin contents are calcium, phosphorus, iron, carotene, thiamine, riboflavin, niacin and vitamin C. Its calorific value is 87.

Parsley contains a glucoside apiin and an essential oil which contain apiol. The fruits contain coumarin.

Healing Power and Curative Properties

Parsley is rich in ascorbic acid and hence is a good blood cleanser. It increases the secretion and discharge of urine and relieves flatulence. Raw parsley juice has some metabolic properties for the normal functioning of the adrenal and thyroid glands.

Digestive Disorders

Parsley aids digestion and helps prevent the formation of gas within the stomach and intestines. It is one of the most popular remedies for indigestion. A couple of sprigs of the fresh herb or a quarter teaspoon of the dried herb can be taken with a glass of water in this condition. As fresh parsley is sometimes rather tough, it should be well masticated.

Genito-Urinary Disorders

According to Dr. R.D. Pope, who has done considerable research on the subject, parsley is "excellent for the genito-urinary tract, being of great assistance in the calculi of the kidneys and bladder, albuminuria, nephritis and other kidney troubles".[1] It has been used as an effective food remedy for dropsy.

High Blood Pressure

The elements in parsley help to maintain the blood vessels, particularly the capillaries and arterial system, in a healthy condition. It is thus very useful in high blood pressure. It may be taken as a beverage by simmering it gently in water for a few minutes, several times daily.

Eye Disorders

Raw parsely juice, mixed with carrot juice, is effective in all ailments connected with the eyes and the optic nerves. It is good for weak eyes, ulceration of the cornea, cataracts, conjunctivitis and opthalmia or sluggishness of the pupil.

Menstrual Disorders

The herb is an effective remedy for scanty menstruation. It

---

1. Dr. S.J. Singh, Food Remedies, 4th edition, published by Nature Cure Council of Medical Research, Lucknow, 1982.

also assists in the regularization of the monthly periods. This action is due to the presence of apiol, a constituent of the female sex hormone—estrogen. Cramps as a result of menstrual irregularities are relieved and frequently corrected by the regular use of parsley juice, specially when combined with beet, carrot and cucumber juices.

Insect Bites and Wounds

Bruised parsley is good as an application to the bites and stings of insects. Likewise, it is very effective when applied on bruised and inflamed joints. It is a most cleansing suppuration when applied to open wounds.

Bad Breath

Parsley is a very effective remedy for bad breath. Boil 2 cups of water with coarsely chopped parsley sprigs and 2 or 3 whole cloves or a quarter tablespoon ground cloves. The mixture has to be stirred frequently while cooling. It is then strained and can be used as a mouthwash or gargle several times a day.

Boils

The herb has also proved beneficial in the treatment of boils. It should be steeped in boiled water till it is soft and juicy. It can be applied to the boils when comfortably hot and wrapped with clean muslin or linen.

Precautions: Raw parsley juice is an extremely potent remedy. It should never be taken in quantities exceeding 60 ml at a time, especially when mixed with a larger quantity of carrot or other raw vegetable juices such as celery, lettuce or spinach.

Other Uses

Parsley can be added freely to salads and soups. Uncooked parsley is palatable and easy to digest when used by itself or cooked with other green vegetables like cabbage or roots. It can also be dried and used. Parsley can be taken as a beverage, simmering it gently for a few minutes and partaking of the water.

Peepal

Botanical Name: *Ficus religiosa*
Indian Name: *Peepal*

Origin, Distribution and Composition

The peepal is one of the best known trees of India. The tree grows to large proportions. It has a hard, cracked and greyish white bark and numerous offshoots. Its leaves are somewhat leathery, broadly oval in shape, which suddenly narrow at the apex and into a long tail.

The peepal is venerated by the Hindus and the Buddhists. The *rishis* of yore meditated under it. It was beneath a peepal that Gautam Buddha attained enlightenment, and that particular tree came to be called *Bodhi*, the 'tree of wisdom'. In the popular Indian folkore, the peepal is considered as the female to the male banyan.

The tree is found wild in the forests on the lower slopes of the Himalayas, Orissa and in Central India. It grows wild in most parts of India, especially on the banks of rivers and lakes.

Healing Power and Curative Properties

The bark and leaves of peepal are useful in many common ailments. Its leaves are laxative and a tonic. They relieve feverish feeling and produce a feeling of coolness. They are also useful in arresting secretion or bleeding—about 50 ml of raw juice of the leaves or 1 teaspoon of powdered dried leaves can be taken with water in such cases.

Heart Diseases

The leaves of the peepal are used in the treatment of heart diseases. They are infused in water at night, distilled the next morning and then stored in white bottles. About 15 mg of this infusion is administered thrice daily. It is highly effective in relieving palpitation of the heart and cardiac weakness.

Constipation

The leaves of the tree are useful in constipation.They should be dried in the shade and powdered. Pills can be prepared by adding the required quantity of a solution of anise and jaggery with water. One pill taken with warm milk at bedtime ensures proper bowel movement the following morning.

Likewise, its fruits can be dried in shade, powdered and mixed with an equal quantity of sugar. This compound in doses of 4 to 6 grams, taken at bedtime with milk, serves the same function.

Dysentery

Its leaves are very effective in treating dysentery. Equal parts of tender leaves, coriander leaves and sugar are chewed slowly to relieve the condition.

Bruises

Its leaves are also useful in bruises and wounds. They are ground fine, mixed with 25 grams of jaggery and made into 8 pills. One pill taken daily with milk can also relieve pain due to injury.

Scrofula

In *Ayurveda*, a peepal grown on a cemented wall, with its roots still in the masonry and not reaching the ground—is a specific for scrofula—a serious disease of the neck, characterised by swollen lymphatic glands of the region. A plaster-like paste prepared by rubbing its root with water can be applied on the glands of the affected people.

Mumps

Peepal leaves are used in the treatment of mumps. They should be smeared with *ghee*, warmed over a fire, and bandaged over the inflamed part to get relief.

Boils

The leaves are also used in boils. A leaf smeared with *ghee* can be bandaged lukewarm on the boil. If there is any pus formation, it will burst, if it is in preliminary stages, the growth will subside.

Other Uses

A popular remedy for excessive urine output amongst jaundice patients is to soak a piece of tender bark of the peepal in water overnight and allow the water to be taken the following morning.

Its fruits dried in shade and powdered are helpful in sexual disorders like spermatorrhoea, nocturnal emissions, and premature ejaculations.

Pepper

Botanical Name: *Piper nigrum*
Indian Name: *Kali mirch*

Origin, Distribution and Composition

Pepper is one of the oldest and most important of all spices. It is known as the "king of spices". The pepper plant is a stout, smooth evergreen creeper, much swollen at its nodes.

Black pepper is the whole dried fruit, while white is the fruit subjected to treatment in water with the mesocarp removed. Both varieties are ground and used in a powdered form.

Pepper was mentioned by Theophrastus in 372-287 B.C. It was used by the ancient Greeks and Romans. By the Middle Ages, pepper had assumed great importance and was used to season food and as a preservative in curing meats. Together with other spices, it helped overcome the odours of bad food.

Pepper is a native of the Western Ghats of India but has now been introduced into most tropical countries.

An analysis of black pepper shows it to consist of moisture 13.2 per cent, protein 11.5 per cent, fat 6.8 per cent, minerals 4.4 per cent, fibre 14.9 per cent and carbohydrates 49.2 per cent, per 100 grams. Its mineral and vitamin contents are calcium, iron, phosphorus, carotene, thiamine, riboflavin and niacin. Its calorific value is 304.

Healing Power and Curative Properties

Black pepper is stimulant, pungent, aromatic, digestive and nervine tonic. Its pungency is due to the resin chavicine, which is most abundant in the mesocarp. Black pepper is useful in relieving flatulence.

Digestive Disorders

Pepper has a stimulating effect on the digestive organs and produces an increased flow of saliva and gastric juices. It is an appetiser and a good home remedy for digestive disorders. Powdered black pepper, thoroughly mixed with malted jaggery, may be taken in the treatment of such conditions. Alternatively, a quarter teaspoon of pepper powder mixed in thin buttermilk can be taken during indigestion or heaviness in the stomach. For better results, an equal part of cumin powder may also be added to the buttermilk.

141

Common Cold

Pepper is beneficial in the treatment of cold and fever. Six pepper seeds finely ground and mixed in a glass of warm water along with 6 pieces of *batasha*—a variety of sugar candy, can be taken for a few nights for good results. In case of acute coryza or cold in the head, 20 grams pepper powder boiled in milk with a pinch of turmeric powder can be used once daily for three days.

Amnesia

A pinch of finely ground pepper mixed with honey taken twice a day is effective in amnesia or dullness of intellect.

Coughs

Pepper is an effective remedy for coughs caused due to throat irritation. Three peppers sucked with a pinch of caraway seeds and a crystal of common salt provides relief.

Impotency

Eating 6 peppers with 4 almonds once daily with milk, is a nerve-tonic and acts as an aphrodisiac especially in an impotent person.

Muscular Pains

As an external application, pepper dilates the superficial vessels and acts as a counter-irritant. A tablespoon of pepper powder fried in sesame oil until it is charred can be applied beneficially as an analgesic liniment for mylagia and rheumatic pains.

Teeth Disorders

Pepper powder and common salt mixture is an excellent dentifrice. Its daily use prevents dental caries, foul breath, bleeding from the gums, painful gums, toothaches and cures the increased sensitiveness of the teeth. A pinch of pepper powder mixed with clove oil can be put in the caries to alleviate toothache.

Pyorrhoea

Pepper is useful in pyorrhoea or pus in the gums. Finely powdered pepper and salt mixture when massaged over the gums relieves inflammation.

Other Uses

Pepper is most widely used as a condiment, its flavour and pungency blending well with most savoury dishes. It is extensively used in pickles, ketchups, sausages and for seasoning dishes.

Poppy Seeds

Botanical Name: *Papaver somniferum*
Indian Name: *Khas-khas*

Origin, Distribution and Composition

Poppy plant is a native of Asia Minor. It was known to the ancient Greeks, and reached India and China by the eighth century. The main areas of cultivation are now in India, China, Asia Minor and the Balkans.

The milky ooze from poppy plant obtained by incision from the unripened capsules and thickened by spontaneous evaporation, is known as opium. Opium is one of the most valuable medicines available in the sap of the plants and if properly administered, can serve as a very useful drug.

Poppy seeds are found in poppy heads. They are recommended in many prescriptions for tonics. The plant is endowed with roots of strong fragrance. It is an erect, annual herb, with smooth surface and latex in all parts.

An analysis of poppy seeds shows them to consist of moisture, protein, fat, fibre and substantial amount of carbohydrates. Its mineral contents are calcium and phosphorus. Its calorific value is 408.

The sap of the plant contains oxalic acid and opium which has 25 alkaloids, the chief being morphine, codeine, thelaine, narcotine, narceine and papaverine.

Healing Power and Curative Properties

Poppy seeds are effective in thirst, fever, inflammation and irritation of the stomach. The root is employed as one of the ingredients in several cooling medicines. An infusion of the root is given as a febrifuge or fever relieving drink—and a powder in bilious complaints. The essence of the root is used as tonic because of its stimulating qualitites. It is believed to check vomiting in cholera.

Insomnia

About 30 grams of milk extracted from the seeds mixed with sugar can be used for treating insomnia. A teaspoon of poppy seed oil taken every night is also very effective.

Dysentery

Here is an easy-to-make home remedy for dysentery. About quarter teaspoon of the powder of poppy seeds are sauted to a golden brown in honey. Taken twice a day, it gives relief from the symptoms. As these seeds have a sedative effect, they should not be take for more than three days continuously.

Pains and Aches

Poppy seeds on the stalks, which have not been slit to produce opium have soporific properties and are used for relieving pain. They can be used beneficially in griping pains after child-birth, colic and pain in the testicles.

Opium is useful in rheumatism, tumours of different kinds, cancers, carbuncles, abscesses, ulcers, leprosy, syphilis or scrofula —that is, tuberculosis of the lymph node in which pain banishes sleep, especially at night. The commencing dose is 6 centigram of the extract. If it is insufficient, upto 18 centigrams may be advised to those who are unaccustomed to opium. Beyond this, it is unsafe to go without any professional advice. This may be combined with 12 or 18 centigrams of camphor. Opium is very effective in spasms of bowels, relieving of pain and irritaition of the bladder caused by stone.

Heat and Burning Sensation

As an external remedy, the poppy plant has many uses. A paste of the root rubbed on the skin can remove burning sensation of the body. A paste of its pulverised roots in water can be used as a cooling agents. It finds use in external application in fevers.

Dry Itch

Poppy seeds ground to paste with lime juice are effective when rubbed on the areas affected by dry itch.

Muscular and Other Pains

Opium is useful as a liniment for soothing both muscular and neuralgic pains. The liniment can be prepared by mixing 90 centigrams of opium in 15 grams of coconut oil. It even soothes painful piles. In painful teeth cavities, a centigram of opium is put into the hollow of the tooth, but the saliva should not be swallowed.

Precautions: Opium can cause great harm if used without proper precautions, or in cases where the person is intolerant to its action or gets upset even with a smallest dose. In such cases, the drug should be avoided.

Infants and young children have poor tolerance to opium and they should be administered only under medical advice. It should be avoided during pregnancy and in kidney diseases.

Rauwolfia

Botanical Name: *Rauwolfia serpentina*
Indian Name: *Sarpagandha*

Origin, Distribution and Composition

Rauwolfia is an erect herb with a smooth stem. The drug consists of the dried roots with their bark intact, preferably collected in autumn from three or four-year-old plants.

Rauwolfia is indigenous to India. The trade name rauwolfia refers to a 16th century German botanist and physician, Leonard Rauwolfia. This plant is believed to have been used in Indian system of medicine for about 4,000 years. It has been mentioned in Charaka's work. Its roots have been valued in India and the Malayan peninsula from ancient times as an antidote for the bites of poisonous reptiles and insects. It is also used as a febrifuge or fever-relieving drug.

This herb was introduced to the modern system of medicine by Dr. Ganpath Sen and Dr. Kartik Chandra Bose, renowned Ayurvedic physicians of Calcutta.[1] Based on their studies they found that the roots contain several alkaloids, the more important being two chemical classes known as the ajmaline and the

---

1. R.N. Chopra, I.C. Chopra, K.L. Handa and L.D. Kapur, Indigenous Drugs of India, 2nd edition reprint, p. 398, Academic Publishers, Calcutta, 1982.

serpentine group. The quantity of the total alkaloids has been estimated to be fairly high in the dried roots. The roots also contain a lot of resin and starch and when incinerated, leave an ash consisting mainly of potassium carbonate, phosphate, silicate and traces of iron and manganese.

Healing Power and Curative Properties

The herb is an effective drug in lowering blood pressure. It is also used to reduce fever. During delivery, it is said to stimulate uterine contractions and promote the expulsion of the foetus. This however, is not corroborated and, maybe regarded as a floklore.

Insanity

The plant is effective in treating insanity. It is popularly known as *pagal-ka-dawa*, a medicine for insanity. It is sold in some parts of India, specifically Bihar and U.P., under this name and is commonly used by practitioners of the indigenous system of medicine. One gram of the powdered root can be taken twice a day with 250 ml of goat's milk, sweetened with sugar candy. Everyone suffering from insanity will not however be benefited by rauwolfia, except those extremely irritable patients with strong physique. Lean, weak and melancholic patients should have their blood pressure examined before the treatment and if found abnormally high, rauwolfia can be tried. As such it is unsuitable for those with a low blood pressure.

Insomnia

The herb is effective in treating insomnia because of its sedative properties. Consequently, the drug is apparently abused by the poorer classes in Bihar, who administer it to infants to induce sleep. The very first dose of rauwolfia enables the patient of a phlegmatic and gouty nature to go to sleep. About 0.60 to 1.25 grams of the powder of its root is mixed with some scented vehicle and taken. It is non-stimulating and should be given in doses of 0.25 grams to the patient at bedtime for sound sleep. A chronic patient should take 0.25 grams, both in the morning and at night before retiring.

High Blood Pressure

Rauwolfia is the best remedy for high blood pressure, and it has been adapted by medical fraternity in most countries, especially American countries. Those alkoloids which have a direct effect on hypertension, have been isolated in it and are widely used by the practitioners of modern medicine. But they have certain unpleasant side effects which the drug taken in its raw form, does not have. Practitioners of the Ayurvedic medicine have preferred to use its root in a powdered form. Half a teaspoon of which taken thrice a day is effective in relieving hypertension.

Hysteria

Rauwolfia is also very effective in treating hysteria. One gram of powdered root can be administered thrice with milk. Treatment should be continued till a complete cure is obtained.

Urticaria

Rauwolfia relieves itching in urticaria. One gram of powdered root can be taken with water.

Rhubarb

Botanical Name: *Rheum emodi*
Indian Name: *Revand chini*

Origin, Distribution and Composition

Rhubarb is a tall perennial herb which has very stout stems and roots with large radical leaves. The dried rhizomes, that is, the underground stems producing roots and leaf shoots of the plant, constitute the drug. The rhizomes should be collected from six or seven year old plants just before the flowering season. The root barks should be retained.

Rhubarb is a native of south eastern Russia. It is one of the oldest recorded herbal drugs, being mentioned in a Chinese herbal remedy dated around 2700 B.C. Rhubarb was introduced in Europe in comparatively recent times. It reached Britain only in the 16th century. It is now cultivated to a limited extent in India and Central Africa.

An analysis of rhubarb stalks shows it to consist substantial amount of moisture, protein, fat, minerals, fibre and carbohydrates. Their mineral and vitamin contents are calcium, phosphorus, iron and vitamin C. Its calorific value is 26.

The rhizomes of rhubarb yield glucoside rhaponticin and

chrysophanic acid. The chief constituents of the herb are antheoquinone derivatives. The roots contain rhein and emodin. Rhizomes also yield an essential oil containing eugenol, a terpene alcohol and a product believed to be methyl heptyl ketone.

Healing Power and Curative Properties

The herb is pungent and bitter. It increases the secretion and discharge of urine.

Constipation

Rhubarb is employed in allopathic medicine largely as a purgative. It also contains tannins and therefore, after purgation, it creates an astringent effect which causes constipation. It is thus suitable only in mild cases of constipation and not in chronic ones.

Diarrhoea

Due to its astringent action, rhubarb can be taken with beneficial results in cases of diarrhoea caused by the presence of any irritating substances in the intestines.

Children's Ailments

Rhubarb is a valuable everyday remedy in ailments of children. It is a safe purgative and also reduces excessive acidity in the digestive tract of children. Sometimes children develop diarrhoea due to excessive consumption of milk which causes putrefaction and consequently increases the acidity in the stomach. Rhubarb expels the putrefied faecal matter simultaneously reduces the acidity. Despite its constipative after effect, the motion stops automatically after the bowels are cleaned. Its dose is one gram for infants upto 2 years old.

Poison Ivy

Rhubarb is one of the effective home remedies for poison ivy. Raw rhubarb rubbed over the area where it itches, gives relief. The treatment is repeated if itching persists.

Other Disorders

Rhubarb is also useful in treating biliousness, lumbago, agitated mind, sore eyes, piles, chronic bronchitis, chronic fever, asthma and coryza, pains and bruises.

Precautions: Rhubarb contains a considrable amount of oxalic acid. Daily use can lead to the formation of stones either in the kidney or the bladder and distressing nervous symptoms.

It should be avoided altogether by those who have a tendency to wounds, gout, rheumatism, epilepsy and other associated diseases with uric acid.

Other Uses

The succulent petioles or leafy stalks are used for pies and sauces.

Rosemary

Botanical Name: *Rosmarinus officinalis*
Indian Name: *Rusmary*

Origin, Distribution and Composition

Rosemary is a sweet scented evergreen shrub which grows upto two metres high. Its leaves are narrow and resemble curved pine needles. They are green on top and grey underneath. The small pale blue flowers grow in little clusters up the stems. Dried leaves of rosemary are used for commercial purposes. Dried herb is brownish green in colour. The leaves have a tea-like fragrance. Crushed rosemary, however, has spicy camphoraceous aroma and a pungent, bitter taste.

Rosemary has long been regarded as the herb for remembrance. Mystically, it symbolises loyalty, love and immortality. It was once believed to strengthen the heart as well as memory.

The Greeks and the Romans prepared a fragrant distilled water from the flowers and inhaled the odour so that the evils were destroyed from the mind and the memory no longer played tricks. In ancient Greece, students preparing for examinations threaded sprigs of rosemary in their locks to induce clear thinking and a good memory.

Rosemary is a native of southern Europe and grows wild on dry rocky hills in the Mediterranean region. It is cultivated across in Yugoslavia, Spain, Portugal, and the U.S.A. In India, it is cultivated in gardens in cool climates for its pleasantly fragrant leaves. It is suitable for cultivation in the temperate Himalayas and Nilgiri hills which have dry to moderately moist climate.

Dried rosemary leaves, on fractional distillation, yield 1 to

2 per cent of a volatile oil which is used in perfumery and medicine. They also contain several acids and other chemical substances. A fraction of phenolic possessing anti-oxidant properties has been isolated from the leaves and its oil.

Healing Power and Curative Properties

Rosemary is an antidote to mental fatigue and forgetfulness. A tea made from the herb is a good natural remedy for bringing added mental agility. It is believed that if the crushed leaves of rosemary are inhaled with the eyes closed, the mind becomes clear as the vapour courses through the brain cells.

Indigestion

The plant has been found useful in atonic dyspepsia, that is, indigestion and stiffness in the stomach. It is specially valuable in the digestion of starchy foods and vegetables like egg-plant and lima beans besides rich meats like pork, beef and lamb.

Flatulence

Its oil is used as an ingredient in rubefacient liniments. Rosemary is formally recognised as a drug in some of the pharmacopoeias. It is mildly irritant and is used to relieve flatulence.

Common Cold

Rosemary oil induces copious perspiration. It can be beneficially mixed in hot water and taken as a drink in colds and chills. The oil is obtained by fractional distillation of the leaves, flowering tops and twigs of the plant. This emulsion is prepeared by mixing oil in hot water. The emulsion is used as a gargle for sore throat. The oil exhibits antibacterial activity.

Rheumatism

The flowering tops and leaves have a camphor-like odour, which induce copious perspiration. They are used for vapour baths in rheumatism.

Other Uses

Heart Stimulant: A few drops of rosemary oil are taken internally as a heart stimulant. A five per cent tincture prepared by mixing oil of rosemary in alcohol, is used as a circulatory and cardiac stimulant.

Dandruff: Shampoos and hair lotions containing the pure

extract of rosemary rejuvenate the scalp and hair while preventing dandruff and premature baldness. A lotion from leafy rosemary branches can be prepared by simmering them in water for 30 minutes before straining and cooling. It can be used as the final hair rinse.

Fresh tender tops are used for garnishing and flavouring cold drinks, pickles, soups, and other foods. Its leaves are used as a condiment. Dried and powdered, they are added to cooked meats, fish, poultry, soups, stews, sauces, garnishings, preserves and jams.

Rough Chaff

Botanical Name: *Achyranthes aspera*
Indian Name: *Chirchita*

Origin, Distribution and Composition

Rough chaff is an erect and stiff annual herb which grows densely upto 50 cm in length. It has numerous branches; almost round and slightly ribbed stem, light green or light pink in colour and covered with short, stiff and slightly rough hair. Its branches have thorns which are pointed downwards. The leaves of the plant are simple, egg-shaped and green. The flowers are small and face downwards. Old flowers are found at the bottom and fresh ones on the upper portion.

The herb occurs in temperate and sub-tropical Himalayas from Kishtwar to Sikkim and Khasi hills at 1200 to 1820 metres, Bihar, Konkan, Nilgiris and Travancore hills. Its seeds and the dried plant are available with grocers and dealers of raw drugs throughout India.

The ash of the herb contains a high proportion of potash and is an antacid. It is an important constituent of alkaline medicine which is useful in counteracting acidity.

Healing Power and Curative Properties

Rough chaff is one of the important herbs used by villagers in preparing mixed greens. The leaves are tasteless but assume a mild bitter taste after cooking. They also have soft cellulose.

151

Asthma

Rough chaff is used to treat asthma. The method prescribed in *Ayurveda* is as follows. The leaves of the plant should be plucked in pitch darkness with no light on the plant at the time of plucking. This is because the presence of light destroys the curative effect of the leaves. After plucking, 25 grams of the leaves are ground with two grams of black pepper on a stone. Six pills are made of the paste which are dried in a dark room the same night. The asthma patient has to take one pill with water on the ninth night of the second half of the lunar month, and continue to follow the procedure for 6 days upto new moon day.

Coughs

The ash of the herb, mixed with honey, is used for coughs. A mixture of the ash and 4 times its weight of water should be allowed to stand for 24 hours. The residue obtained by evaporating the supernatant or upper layers of the liquid is the well-known Ayurvedic prepartion *aghada khara*. It is taken in doses of 6 to 12 centigrams for relieving coughs.

Spleen Enlargement

The herb is specific for spleen enlargement. The powder of the plant is used in 25 gram doses twice daily with a little beaten curd. This brings good results in 3 or 4 weeks.

Cholera

The powdered root of the herb is very useful in cholera. About 6 grams of the powder should be mixed with water and taken.

Renal Dropsy

A decoction of the plant is beneficial in renal dropsy as it increases the secretion and discharge of urine. This decoction is prepared by boiling 60 grams of the plant in 150 ml of water for 20 to 30 minutes. About 30 to 60 grams of this strained mixture should be taken twice or thrice daily.

Stomach Disorders

The juice of the leaves is valuable in stomach disorders like stomach ache, bowel complaints and piles. A decoction of the powdered leaves, mixed with honey or sugar candy is useful in the early stages of diarrhoea and dysentery.

Menorrhagia

This is a condition of excessive menstrual bleeding. The drug is useful in arresting secretion or bleeding. It is therefore valuable in abnormally excessive menstruation. An infusion of the herb should be used in treating this condition.

Skin Problems

The leaves of rough chaff are useful in cuts and wounds from sharp-edged weapons like knives and blades. Juice of a few leaves of the plant is used to thoroughly soak the wound. A leaf should be wrapped and bandaged over it. It heals within a day or two with a single application. An ointment made of the ash of the herb with orpiment is used for clearing warts and ulcers.

Eye Disorders

The root of the herb is useful for eye-disorders. A paste of the roots with water can be applied beneficially in opthalmia and opacity of the cornea.

Insect Bites

A paste of the leaves made with water has proved effective in treating bites of poisonous insects, wasps, bees etc. It should be applied externally over the affected parts.

Precautions: It is advisable for pregnant women to take the juice of the herb in small doses, as large doses may hasten labour pains or cause abortion.

Other Uses

Easy Delivery: Rough chaff seeds are useful in facilitating easy and painless delivery. The seeds are ground well in water to prepare a fine paste, and applied on the navel, pubis and vulva.

Sage

Botanical Name: *Salvia officinalis*
Indian Name: *Salvia or sefakuss*

Origin, Distribution and Composition

Sage is an evergreen woody-stemmed shrub which grows up to 60 cms high. It has greyish green stalked slender leaves, rough in texture. The flowers are purplish blue. The dried herb is grey, tinged with green. It has strong spicy aroma and a slightly bitter and astringent taste.

It has a centuries-old reputation of exerting a beneficial influence on the brain, nerves, eyes and glands. Gerard testified the effectiveness of the herb for "quickening the senses and memory, strengthening the sinews and restoring health to those suffering from palsies and trembling of limbs".[1]

Sage originated in the Mediterranean countries but is now cultivated in Europe, Canada and the United States. In India, its cultivation in gardens has been tried in Jammu for its essential oil. The plants are reported to have done well and the quality of the oil obtained is comparable to that of foreign origin.

Sage contains a volatile oil, resin, tannin and a bitter principle. The oil is composed of camphor, salvene, cineol and pinene. The fresh leaves provide appreciable amounts of vitamin A and C.

Healing Power and Curative Properties

Sage has always played a great part in the history of botanic medicine. The Chinese adage 'sage for old age' sums up its healthful qualities. It has a reputation to retard old age, restore energy and aid digestion. In pharmaceutical writings, sage is listed among the natural antiseptics.

Failing Memory

Sage is considered very useful in failing memory. The herb acts on the cortex of the brain thereby eliminating mental exhaustion and improving concentration.

---

1. Dr. S.J. Singh, *Food Remedies*, 4th edition, p. 175, Nature Cure Council of Medical Research, Lucknow, 1982.

Stress

Tea prepared from sage leaves is beneficial in coping with stress. It can be prepared by pouring a cup of boiling water over 1 teaspoon of dried sage leaves with lid on. It should be infused for few minutes before straining and sweetening with honey, if desired. In case of fresh leaves, a tablespoon of chopped sage leaves can be used and tea prepared similarly.

Infections

Leafy sprigs of sage were among the strewing herbs spread on the floors of old manors, for it was believed to be an antiseptic to gaurd against plague and other infections.

Premature Greying of Hair

The herb is useful in preventing grey hair if blended in hair tonics.

Sore Throat

Sage is known for its healing action on the throat and mouth. Gargles and mouthwashes use it as the principal ingredient. Leaves rubbed on the teeth regularly help to keep them sparkling white and strengthen the gums.

To treat sore throat, half a litre of boiling water should be poured on a handful of sage leaves. When moderately cool, a little vinegar and honey should be added. This mixture should be used as a gargle. While gargling, a teaspoon of this mixture can also be taken internally.

Other Uses

Sage is one of the most popular herbs used in culinary preparations in the west. It helps counteract the harmful richness of foods like pork, goose, duck and oily fish. It also combines well with dairy foods, bean and pea soups. Dried and powdered leaves are mixed with cooked vegetables and sprinkled on cheese dishes. Fresh sage leaves are used in salads and sandwiches.

Sandalwood

Botanical Name: *Santalum album*
Indian Name: *Chandan*

Origin, Distribution and Composition

Sandalwood is a medium-sized evergreen tree with almost drooping branches, dark rough bark and scented mature wood. It has opposite leaves, shining on the upper surface, with small dull purplish flowers in small bunches and roundish, purple-black succulent fruits. Its trade name sandalwood is based on its Indian name.

Sandalwood is believed to be indigenous to India. It is cultivated in Karnataka, Coorg, Coimbatore and the southern parts of Tamil Nadu. It also grows wild.

Sandalwood occupies a very important place in Hindu religious rituals. The Parsis use it for the fire in their temples. Its wood was highly prized during ancient India and China owing to its sweet odour. This tree finds a mention in the earliest Sanskrit and Chinese literature.

Sandalwood yields an essential oil which contains santaloe.

Healing Power and Curative Properties

Both the sandalwood, and the essential oil obtained after fractional distillation, have been used in *Ayurveda* for many centuries. The wood is bitter, sedative, cooling and a cardiac tonic. It is useful in arresting secretion or bleeding and in promoting the flow of urine. Moreover, sandalwood oil is a stimulant and an antiseptic. It has a soothing effect on the skin and mucous membranes.

Genito-Urinary Disorders

Sandalwood powder mixed with milk or made into pills, as also sandalwood oil, is considered beneficial in the treatment of gonorrhoea. Sandalwood oil is used in treating, dysuria (painful and difficult urination) and cystitis (inflammation of the bladder). It is taken in doses of five drops in the beginning and gradually increased to 10 to 30 drops. Its efficacy can be increased by the addition of *ajwain* water or infusion of ginger.

Gastric Irritability

Sandalwood is valuable in gastric irritability. About

156

22 grams of a watery emulsion of the wood mixed with sugar, honey and rice water, should be administered in the treatment of such a condition.

Dysentery

Sandalwood is also beneficial in the treatment of dysentery. It should be administered as for gastric irritability.

Prickly Heat

Sandalwood paste is a popular household remedy for prickly heat. It prevents excessive sweating and heals inflamed skin. Dry sandalwood powder can be mixed in rose water and applied over parts where there is profuse sweating.

Skin Diseases

An emulsion or a paste of the wood is a cooling dressing in inflammatory and eruptive skin diseases such as erysipelas, an inflammatory disease of the face, and prurigo, an itchy eruption. The oil is useful for scabies too. This oil mixed with twice its quantity of mustard oil is used for removing pimples. In summer, regular application of sandalwood paste on the body, especially for children, has a refreshing effect, which heals any tiny infected spots.

Fever

Sandalwood paste applied on the temple relieves headache and brings down the temperature in fevers.

Saussurea

Botanical Name: *Saussurea lappa*
Indian Name: *Kuth*

Origin, Distribution and Composition

Saussurea, known as castus in English, is a tall, stout herb having an annual stem and perennial roots. It has very large heart-shaped leaves, bluish, bluish-purple or almost black flowers and hairy fruits. The dried roots of the plant constitute the drug.

Saussurea is indigenous to India. It occurs in Kashmir and adjoining areas at altitudes ranging from 2,500 to 4,000 metres above the sea level.

The roots of the plant contain an essential oil, alkaloid saussurine and a bitter resin. The resinoid on distillation with superheated steam under reduced pressure yields an essential oil[1]. However, the essential oil contains terpenes, aplotaxene and sesquiterpenes.

Healing Power and Curative Properties

The plant is well-known both in the Ayurvedic and Tibbi medicine. The root has a pungent taste and a peculiar fragrance. It is a tonic, aphrodisiac, antiseptic and a stimulant. It strengthens functioning of the stomach and promotes its action. It is helpful in arresting secretion or bleeding.

The essential oil has antiseptic and disinfectant properties. It relaxes the involuntary muscle tissues and serves as a cardiac stimulant. It relieves flatulences and is a diuretic. It is also useful in removing catarrhal matter and phlegm from the bronchial tubes.

Respiratory Disorders

Saussurea is beneficial in the treatment of respiratory disorders like bronchitis, asthma and cough, especially controlling attacks of bronchial asthma. The combined action of the essential oil and the alkaloid in the root restrict the paroxysms. The alkaloid saussurine has a depressant action on the vagus centre in the medulla, which supplies motor nerve fibre, as well as on the involuntary muscle fibres of the broncholes and gastrointestinal tract. It produces a slight but persistent rise in blood pressure and increases the force of contraction and amplitude of the ventricles. The essential oil not only relaxes the bronchial muscle, but also has a marked expectorant action which relieves turgescene of the mucosa. It, however, does not produce a permanent cure unless the causal factors are investigated into and removed.

Cholera

This powerful aromatic stimulant is also useful in cholera. An infusion made of 3 grams of fresh saussurea, 1 gram of cardamom and 120 ml of water can be administered in

---

1. R.N. Chopra, S.L. Nayar and I.C. Chopra, *Glossary of Indian Medicinal Plants*, p.222, CSIR, New Delhi.

30 gram doses every half an hour in treating this condition. The essential oil in the herb produces reflex inhibition by its stimulating properties. It helps in controlling the disease. It is an irritant and has a strong penetrating and persistent odour and taste. The depressant action of the drug on the brain helps in relieving the spasm.

Ulcer

Saussurea is useful for severe ulcerations. The dried and powdered root is the principal ingredient in any astringent and stimulant ointment.

Premature Greying of Hair

The herb prevents premature greying of hair. The dried and powdered root can be used as hair wash.

Other Uses

Aphrodisiac: In the indigenous medicine in India, saussurea is used as tonic and as an aphrodisiac. During its passage through the urethra the essential oil excreted in the urine produces a certain amount of irritation, acting as a stimulant.

The root forms a very valuable raw material for producing an expensive perfume, closely resembling the violet perfume.

Tamarind

Botanical Name: *Tamarindus indica*
Indian Name: *Imli*

Origin, Distribution and Composition

Tamarind is a large, handsome, symmetrical spreading tree. It has small compound leaves, yellowish flowers with reddish streaks and fleshy, brown fruits. The seeds are dark brown and shiny. The fleshy fibrous pulp of the fruit is acidic.

Tamarind was an important item of diet of sailors in olden times as its acid and sugar content helped them to offset their starchy diet.

Tamarind is a native of Africa but is now grown in most tropical countries.

An analysis of tamarind pulp shows it to consist of moisture

20.9 per cent, protein 3.1 per cent, fat 0.1 per cent, minerals 2.9 per cent, fibre 5.6 per cent and carbohydrates 67.4 per cent. Its mineral and vitamin contents are calcium, phosphorus, iron, carotene, riboflavin, niacin and vitamin C. Its calorific value is 283.

The pulp contains tartaric and other acids, sugars like invert—a broken-up starch, and pectin. The pectin present in the pulp is of good quality.

Healing Power and Curative Properties

The whole plant has medicinal virtues. Its leaves are cooling and antibilious, while the bark is an astringent, a tonic and reduces fever. The fruit pulp is digestive, antiflatulent, cooling, laxative and antiseptic. Its seeds are also astringent.

Digestive Disorders

Pulp of the ripe fruit is beneficial in the treatment of bilious vomiting, flatulence and indigestion. It is also useful in constipation. An infusion of the pulp prepared by softening it in water, is particularly useful for loss of appetite and lack of inclination for food intake. For better results, black pepper, cloves, cardamoms and camphor may be added to taste, to this infusion after straining. The ash obtained by heating the bark with salt in an earthen vessel can also be given in 6 to 12 centigram doses for colic and indigestion with beneficial results.

Scurvy

Tamarind pulp, being rich in vitamin C, is valuable in preventing and curing scurvy. It is significant that tamarind does not lose its antiscorbutic property on drying as in case of other fruits and vegetables.

Common Cold

Tamarind-pepper *rasam*, a clear soup—is considered an effective home remedy for colds in South India. It is prepared by boiling a very dilute tamarind water in a teaspoon of hot *ghee* and half a teaspoon of black pepper powder for a few minutes. This steaming hot *rasam* has a flushing effect. As one takes it, the nose and eyes water and the nasal blockage is cleared.

Fevers

The pulp of tamarind fruit is useful in treating fevers. It is generally taken in 15 gram doses. A *sherbet* made by boiling 30 grams of the pulp in half a litre of milk with the addition of a few dates, cloves, sugar and cardamoms and a little camphor is effective in fevers.

Dysentery

The tamarind milk drink, as suggested for fevers, is also very helpful in treating dysentery. Pulverised seeds taken in doses of 6.25 decigrams, with an equal quantity of cumin and sugar, twice or thrice a day, are also useful.

Burns

The tender leaves of tamarind tree are a useful remedy for treating burns. They are put into a pot, covered and warmed over the fire. The burnt ones are finely powdered and sieved to remove any gritty particles. This is mixed in gingelly *(til)* oil and applied over the burnt part. The wound gets healed within a few days. Its leaves prevent oedema and help in the growth of healthy, normal skin. The oil keeps the affected part well protected against moisture and entry of harmful germs.

Inflammation of Joints

Crushed with water and made into a poultice, the leaves are applied on inflamed joints and ankles. It reduces swelling and pain.

Sore Throat

Gargle of tamarind water is beneficial in the treatment of sore throat. The potion should be prepared by boiling tamarind in water. A powder of the dry leaves can also be beneficially used as a gargle for sore throat. An infusion, of the bark is equally useful for this purpose.

Other Uses

Ripe fruit or tamarind pulp is widely used in culinary preparations, notably *sambhar, rasam* curries and *chutney* in South India.

Trailing Eclipta

Botanical Name: *Eclipta alba*
Indian Name: *Bhangra*

Origin, Distribution and Composition

Trailing eclipta is a small, erect or prostrate, many branched and a coarsely haired annual herb. It grows upto 30 cms in height. It has a round, feeble stem, simple ecliptic and hairy leaves, variable in shape, bright dark green in colour with very small flowers, called florets. Its small, black seeds resemble mustard seeds. Trailing eclipta is indigenous to India and grows as a common weed.

The herb contains alkaloid ecliptine. It also contains alkaloid nicotene and resin. The leaves have more of water and soft cellulose content.

Healing Power and Curative Properties

The fresh plant, leaves and roots are all used for medicinal purposes. The fresh plant and the leaves are tonic. They correct the disordered processes of nutrition and restore the normal function of the system. They also facilitate secretion or excretion by opening the natural passage and pores of the body like of the skin. The roots and leaves of the plant also promote the flow of bile. The leaves have a slighly bitter and acrid taste. It is advisable not to take the leaves alone but to mix them with other bland leaves or some other medium.

Liver and Spleen Disorders

Trailing eclipta is useful in the enlargement of liver and spleen. It is also useful in other liver disorders. A decoction of the herb is taken in doses of 1 teaspoon twice a day. The leaves of the plant can also be used for these disorders and jaundice. One teaspoon of the juice can be mixed with an aromatic such as cardamon and cinnamon. For catarrhal jaundice accompanied with discharge of mucus from the mucous membranes of the intestine, a large pill of fresh leaves, mixed with a few crushed pepper corns, is taken with curd early in the morning for about a week.

Fevers

The drug has the property to relieve feverishness and

produce a feeling of coolness. The fresh juice of the plant should be taken in doses of 2 to 8 ml. The juice of the leaves in combination with cardamom and cinnamon can be taken in fevers in doses of 1 teaspoon.

Catarrh in Babies

The juice of the plant is useful for newborn babies suffering from catarrh. Two drops of the juice mixed with honey is given. The juice of the leaves can also be used for this purpose in doses of 2 drops mixed with 8 drops of honey.

Uterine Haemorrhages

The leaves of the plant are useful in uterine haemorrhages or bleeding. A decoction of the leaves can be taken in doses of 60 to 120 ml, twice a day.

Skin Disorders

Trailing eclipta is good for glandular swellings, elephantiasis and other skin diseases. A paste of the herb mixed with sesame (*til*) oil is applied externally over the affected parts. A paste of the leaves is also applied to chronic glandular swellings, skin diseases and to wounds as a styptic or astringent. The juice of the leaves can be used beneficially for cleaning and healing sores.

Premature Greying of Hair

For premature greying of hair, two parts of the herb, one part of black sesame seeds and one part of Indian gooseberry (*amla*) are finely powdered. One teaspoon of this powder is taken with milk and sugar twice daily for treating this disorder.

Other Uses

Hair Growth: The fresh juice of the leaves is useful in promoting growth of hair. The juice should be rubbed into the scalp for this purpose.

Turmeric

Botanical Name: *Curcuma longa*
Indian Name: *Haldi*

Origin, Distribution and Composition

Turmeric is a perennial herb, 60 to 90 cms high. It has short stem and raised or lifted branches. The rhizomes, or underground stems are short and thick and constitute commercial turmeric. It is an important common flavouring spice of daily use. In India, it is used in the same way as saffron.

Turmeric has been mentioned in early Sanskrit works. It has been used by the Ayurvedic and Unani practitioners in India since ancient times. It was prescribed by them as a drug to strengthen the stomach, promote its action, as a tonic and as a blood purifier.

Turmeric is a native of Southern or South-eastern Asia. It has been grown in India from ancient times. It seems to have reached China before the seventh century A.D. Turmeric spread early throughout the East Indies and was carried eastwards across the Pacific by Polynesians to Hawai and Easter Island.

An analysis of turmeric shows it to consist of moisture 13.1 per cent, protein 6.3 per cent, fat 5.1 per cent, minerals 3.5 per cent, fibre 2.6 per cent and carbohydrates 69.4 per cent. Its mineral and vitamin contents are, calcium, phosphorus, iron, carotene, thiamine and niacin. Its calorific value is 349.

Turmeric contains curcumin and an essential oil. Dry rhizomes yield 5.8 per cent essential oil, while the fresh ones yield 0.24 per cent oil containing zingiberine. Ketone and alcohol are obtained on volatile distillation.

Healing Power and Curative Properties

Turmeric has many medicinal virtues. The rhizome is aromatic, stimulant and a tonic. It is useful in relieving flatulence. It corrects the disordered processes of nutrition and restores the normal function of the system. It is also useful in curing periodic attacks of hysteria and convulsions.

Intestinal Disorders

Turmeric is a very useful intestinal antiseptic. The rhizome, its juice or dry powder, mixed in butter milk or plain water, is highly beneficial in intestinal problems, especially chronic diarrhoea. It also helps prevent flatulence.

Worms

About 20 drops of the juice of raw turmeric, mixed with a pinch of salt, taken first thing in the morning daily, is considered an effective remedy for expelling worms.

Anaemia

Turmeric, being rich in iron, is valuable in anaemia. A teaspoon of raw turmeric juice, mixed with honey, is taken everyday in the treatment of this condition.

Measles

The herb is beneficial in the treatment of measles. Turmeric roots are dried in the sun and ground to a fine powder. This, mixed with a few drops of honey and the juice of few bitter gourd leaves, can be taken by those suffering from measles.

Asthma

Turmeric is an effective household remedy for bronchial asthma. A teaspoon of turmeric powder with a glass of milk, twice or thrice daily is very effective. It acts best on an empty stomach.

Cough and Cold

Turmeric, with its antiseptic properties, is an effective remedy for chronic cough and throat irritations. Half a teaspoon of fresh turmeric powder, mixed in 30 ml of warm milk is very effective in these conditions. To perpare this, milk is poured on a hot ladle with turmeric in it and boiled over a slow fire. In case of a running cold, smoke from burning turmeric can be inhaled. This increases the discharge from the nose and brings quicker relief.

Turmeric, in combination with caraway seeds or *ajwain,* is useful for colds in infants and children. A teaspoon of turmeric powder and quarter teaspoon of *ajwain* are added to boiling water which is then cooled. About 30 ml of this decoction, sweetened with honey, may be taken thrice a day in treating such conditions.

Sprains

For treating sprains or the swellings caused by sprains, turmeric paste mixed with lime and salt can be applied with beneficial results.

Boils

An application of turmeric powder to boils speeds up the healing process. In case of fresh boils, a few dry roots of turmeric are roasted and the ashes dissolved in a cupful of water and applied over the affected portion. This solution enables the boils to ripen and burst.

Skin Disorders

Turmeric is very effective in the treatment of skin diseases like ringworm and scabies. In such cases, the juice of raw turmeric is externally applied to the affected parts. Simultaneously, turmeric juice, mixed with honey, should be taken orally.

Sore Eyes

Turmeric powder is useful in soreness of the eyes. About 6 grams of this powder is boiled in about half a litre of water till it is reduced to half. A few drops of this water put in the affected eyes, three or four times a day, give relief.

Other Uses

Turmeric is an indispensable culinary ingredient. It imparts a musky flavour and yellow colour to curries. It is also used as a colouring matter in pharmacy, confectionery and food industries.

Turpeth

Botanical Name: *Operculina turpethum*
Indian Name: *Nisoth or Pithori*

Origin, Distribution and Composition

Turpeth, also known as Indian jalap, is a large, stout twining perennial herb with sap. It has a many branched root and quadrangular, winged stems. Its leaves are egg-shaped and heart-shaped. Its white flowers are funnel-shaped in bunches. Its fruits are roundish with usually fourseeds to each. The herb is also called as Indian rhubarb or Indian jalap because of its purgative characteristic.

The dried roots of the plant constitute the drug. There are

two varieties of this plant, with either white or black tuberous roots. The roots of the white variety has to be used. The trade name is based on its scientific name.

The bark of the plant contains a glycosidic resin, which has ether insoluble glycoside turpethein and two ether soluble glycosides. Besides, it also contains a small amount of volatile oil, glucose and fructose.

Healing Power and Curative Properties

Turpeth has long been used in India as a cathartic, that is, a drug which induces active movement of the bowels, but it was officially recognised in the list of Indian Pharmacopoeia only in 1946. Only the dried roots of the white variety with its bark intact finds its place there.

Chronic Constipation

Turpeth is used as a purgative. It has almost the same properties as the true jalap, botanically known as *exogonium purga* and can be used with advantage as its substitute. It is superior to the herb rhubarb. Its powdered roots are used as a purgative and to relieve any chronic constipation.

Arthritis

The drug is beneficial in treating rheumatic and paralytic diseases. A single dose of 3 to 4 grams should be taken daily.

Dropsy

Turpeth is a valuable drug in the treatment of dropsical affections. The tuberous roots in doses of 2 to 4 grams mixed with chebulic myroblan *(harad)* are especially beneficial in such disorders.

Gout

For the treatment of gout, it is administered in the same way as for dropsical affections.

Jaundice

In *Ayurveda*, turpeth is considered to be one of the two major drugs with which the treatment of jaundice should start, the other drug being *kutuki*. One or two teaspoon of the powder of each of the two drugs may be administered with hot water twice daily.

Other Diseases

Turpeth is also effective for other diseases like melancholia, leprosy, enlargement of spleen and paralysis. Its efficacy increases, when mixed with chebulic myroblan.

Vasaka

Botanical Name: *Adhatoda vasica*
Indian Name: *Adusa*

Origin, Distribution and Composition

Vasaka, also called Malabar nut tree, is well known throughout India. It is tall, with several branches, dense, and an evergreen shrub. Leaves are large and lance-shaped. It has capsular four-seeded fruits. The flowers are either white or purple in colour. Its trade name vasaka is based on Sanskrit name.

Vasaka is indigenous to India. It grows all over the plains of India and in the lower Himalayan ranges.

The leaves contain an alkaloid vasicine besides an essential oil.

Healing Power and Curative Properties

The leaves, roots and the flowers are extensively used in indigenous medicine as a remedy for cold, cough, bronchitis and asthma.

Bronchitis and Asthma

In acute stages of bronchitis it gives unfailing relief, especially where the sputum is thick and sticky. It liquifies the sputum so that it is brought up more easily. For relief in asthma, the dried leaves should be smoked.

Tuberculosis

In *Ayurveda*, a preparation made from vasaka flowers, known as *gulkand* is used to treat tuberculosis. A few fresh petals of vasaka flowers should be bruised and put in a pot of china clay. Some sugar crystals are added and the jar kept in the sun. It should be stirred every morning and evening. The preserve is ready for use in about a month.

Even the juice from its leaves is useful in treating tuberculosis. About 30 ml of the juice is taken thrice a day with honey. It relieves the irritable cough by its soothing action on the nerve and by liquefying the sputum, which makes expectoration easier. U.C. Dutt says, "the medicine was considered so serviceable in phthisis (severe tuberculosis of the lungs) that it was said, no man suffering from this disease need despair as long as the vasaka plant exists".[1]

Coughs

For coughs, 7 leaves of the plant are boiled in water, strained and mixed with 24 grams of honey. This decoction provides relief. Similarly a confection of vasaka flowers eaten in doses of 12 grams twice daily relieves cough. About 60 grams of flowers and 180 grams of jaggery should be mixed for preparing this confection.

Intestinal Worms

Its leaves, bark, the root-bark, the fruit and flowers are useful in the removal of intestinal parasites. The decoction of its root and bark in doses of 30 grams twice or thrice a day for 3 days can be given for this purpose. The juice of its fresh leaves can also be used in doses of a teaspoon thrice a day for 3 days.

Diarrhoea and Dysentery

The juice from its leaves should be given in doses of 2 to 4 grams in treating diarrhoea and dysentery.

Skin Diseases

A poultice of its leaves can be applied with beneficial results over fresh wounds, rheumatic joints and inflammatory swellings. A warm decoction of its leaves is useful in treating scabies and other skin diseases.

Methods for Uses and Dosages : The drug vasaka is often taken in the form of juice extracted from its leaves, mixed with ginger or honey, in doses of 15 to 30. The leaves can be made into a decoction or the dried leaves can be given in powder form in doses of 2 grams. Both the decoction and powder are

---

1. R.N. Chopra, I.C. Chopra, K.L. Handa and L.D. Kapur, Indigenous Drugs of India, 2nd edition reprint, Academic Publishers, Calcutta, 1982.

constituents of many preparations used in the Ayurvedic medicine for various affections of the respiratory tract. The root and the bark have the same medicinal uses as the leaves. A decoction of the bark is given in 30 to 60 ml doses and the powdered root-bark in 0.75 to 2 grams doses.

Watercress

Botanical Name: *Nasturtium officinale*
Indian Name: *Jal-halim or Jal-kumbhi*

Origin, Distribution and Composition

The watercress is a perennial, aquatic herb, with hollow angular stems, and many branches. It has dark green, shining leaves divided into several leaflets. It has a pleasant and pungent flavour and is used in salads.

The Greeks regarded watercress as a psychic stimulant and the Romans used it with vinegar as a remedy for mental disorders. Old English physicians recommended its use as a remedy for headaches and biliousness.

Watercress is a native of Europe. It is widely distributed in a wild state in Great Britain, South and Central Europe and Western Asia. This plant is now cultivated in Malaysia, Indonesia, Hawaii, West Indies and East Africa and grows wild in the Himalayas.

Watercress contains all the essential vitamins and is rich in alkaline elements. An analysis of this vegetable shows it to consist of moisture, protein, fat and carbohydrates. Its mineral and vitamin contents are calcium, phosphorus, magnesium, iron, sodium, potassium, vitamins A and C, thiamine, riboflavin and niacin. Its calorific value is 19. The herb also contains nicotinamide, a glucoside, gluconasturtin and a volatile oil.

Healing Power and Curative Properties

Watercress has a cooling effect on the body and, aids digestion. Hippocrates described it as a stimulant and expectorant.

Anaemia

As a rich source of iron, watercress is beneficial in the

treatment of anaemia. A cup of its fresh juice with a teaspoon of lime juice and a pinch of commonsalt can be taken every morning for a month in the treatment of this condition.

Asthma

The herb is considered an excellent food remedy for chest troubles. It has been found effective in treating asthma and cough as it facilitates expectoration.

Disorders of the Thyroid Gland

Watercress is one of the best sources of iodine which is very important to correct the functioning of the thyroid gland. Its regular use is highly beneficial in the prevention and treatment of thyroid gland disorders.

Piles

A combined juice of watercress, carrot, spinach and turnip leaves is effective in dissolving the coagulated blood fibrin in piles. About a litre of this if taken daily it cures this condition within 2 to 6 months. However, all white flour, sugar products and meat have to be eliminated from the diet.

Skin Disorders

A paste made of seeds and water, can be applied in skin diseases caused by the impurities of blood. Bruised seeds, mixed with lime juice and spread on linen, can be applied with beneficial results in case of internal inflammation and rheumatic pains. The seed is also effective as a rubefacient—a pain relieving ointment.

Precautions: The juice extracted from watercress is exceedingly rich in sulphur, which represents more than one third of all the other combined mineral elements and salts present in it. It is, however, a very powerful intestinal cleanser. It should, therefore, never be taken by itself but always in combination with other juices.

Other Uses

Dietary Deficiencies: Dr. Harold Scurfield, an eminent British physician has advocated the greater use of watercress among urbanites on the plea that it probably contains all the vitamins which are likely to compensate dietary deficiencies caused by urbanisation.[1]

Malnutrition: Watercress is good for malnutrition. Dr. S. Monckton Copeman, formerly of the Ministry of Health in England, says, "In many instances, excellent results, especially in the case of ill-nourished children, have been found to follow on the addition of watercress to their ordinary food.[2]

Pregnancy and Lactation: The use of watercress is very beneficial during pregnancy and lactation. An invigorating and nutritious tonic is prepared by boiling the seeds in milk to get a thin, soft mass and adding sugar or jaggery, to it. This tonic removes the imminent general debility during pregnancy. It also increases the secretion of milk in nursing mothers.

Hiccups: An emulsion made by soaking the seeds in water is taken as a drink at frequent intervals to relieve hiccups.

Watercress is mostly used as vegetable. Its rich green leaves make an excellent salad. The flowers of the plant are also palatable.

Winter Cherry

Botanical Name: *Withania somnifera*
Indian Name: *Ashvagandha or Akri*

Origin, Distribution and Composition

Winter cherry is a small or middle-sized, erect shrub, growing upto 1.5 metres tall. Its stems and branches are covered with minute star-shaped hairs. It has egg-shaped, hairy leaves upto 10 cms long, small, pale green flowers in clusters of about 25; and smooth, spherical, red fruits with yellow seeds. Its trade name *ashvagandha* is based on its Indian name.

Winter cherry is indigenous to India. It is also found in Afganistan, Pakistan and Sri Lanka.

The herb contains an alkaloid somniferine. Its roots contain traces of an essential oil. The water soluble portion of root

---

1. Dr. S.J. Singh, Food Remedies, 4th edition, p. 204, Nature Cure Council of Medical Research, Lucknow, 1982.

2. Ibid, p. 205.

extract contains indefinite amorphous substances and a quantity of sugar. The water soluble extract consists chiefly of a black resin, which contains,besides other constituents, a mixture of some fatty acids.It also contains potassium nitrate, tannin, colouring matter, glucose and some alkaloids.

Healing Power and Curative Properties

The shrub as a whole is employed for several medicinal applications for its hypnotic and sedative properties. It promotes libido. The root of the plant is a tonic and stimulant. It increases the secretion and discharge of urine and also other forms of secretion or excretion by opening the natural pores of the body. Recent experiments have shown that its roots and leaves possess antibiotic and antibacterial properties.

Digestive Disorders

The root of the plant is used for treating digestive disorders like dyspepsia and loss of appetite. It corrects the disordered processes of nutrition and restores the normalcy in the system.

General Debility

Its root finds its use in treating general debility. It is taken in 2 gram doses for this purpose.

Rheumatism

The root is effective in the treatment of rheumatic affections. It should be taken in 3 gram doses in treating this condition.

Tuberculosis

The root finds its efficacy in treatment of tuberculosis. A decoction of the root is used with long pepper and honey.This decoction is also beneficial in the treatment of scrofula, that is, tuberculosis of lymph glands, especially in the neck.

Insomnia

The root is also a narcotic, inducing deep sleep and hence beneficial in treating insomnia.

Cold and Cough·

Winter cherry is beneficial in the treatment of chest diseases such as cough and cold. The root can be taken either in the form of powder in 3 gram doses or in the form of decoction. Berries and seeds can also be taken for chest complaints with beneficial results.

Women's Diseases

The herb helps to cure female sterility. Powder of the roots in 6 gram doses can be taken with milk for 5 to 6 successive nights after menstruation.

Skin Disorders

The leaves of the plant are beneficial in treating several skin disorders. Fomentation of the leaves is good for boils and swollen hands and feet. A paste of the leaves is locally applied to kill lice infesting the body and on carbuncles (painful swelling inside the skin) and syphilitic sores. An ointment prepared by boiling the leaves in fat such as *ghee* can be applied in case of bedsores and wounds. A paste made of its roots and leaves is also a useful application over carbuncles, ulcers and swellings.

Sore Eyes

For sore eyes, a fomentation of the leaves can be applied to get relief.

Precautions: The drug possesses properties that can abort a foetus and hence must be avoided by pregnant women.

Other Uses

Aphrodisiac: Two to four grams of the root with milk or *ghee* can be taken as an aphrodisiac to enhance libido. The drug is beneficial in the treatment of spermatorrhoea or involuntary ejaulation. Two to four grams of the powdered root can also be taken daily with sugar, honey, long pepper and *ghee* in the treatment of these conditions.

Wood Apple

Botanical Name: *Feronia limonida*
Indian Name: *Kaith*

Origin, Distribution and Composition

Wood apple, is a whitish spherical fruit, with a hard woody pericarp and aromatic pulp. The tree is spiny with feather-like leaves and reddish flowers. The surface of the fruits and branches is very rough and covered with a white bloom.

Wood apple is indigenous to South India. It is also cultivated in tropical Asia.

Wood apple consists of moisture 64.2 per cent, protein 7.1 per cent, fat 3.7 per cent, minerals 1.9 per cent, fibre 5.0 per cent and carbohydrates 18.1 per cent per 100 grams. Its mineral and vitamin contents are calcium, phosphorus, iron, carotene, thiamine, riboflavin, niacin and vitamin. Its calorific value is 134.

Wood apple is rich in oxalic, malic citric acid and a concentrated tannic acid. The leaves yield an essential oil.

Healing Power and Curative Properties

The pulp of the raw fruit is useful in arresting secretion or bleeding. The ripe fruit is refreshing, aromatic, digestive and a tonic. It is useful in preventing and curing scurvy and in relieving flatulence. Its leaves are not only aromatic but also possess some astringent and carminative properties. The gum that the stem exudes has a soothing effect on the skin and mucous membranes.

Digestive Disorders

Mashed seedless pulp of the raw fruit is beneficial in the treatment of dysentery, diarrhoea and piles. The pulp of the ripe fruit, mixed with cardamom, honey and cumin seeds, is effective for indigestion, diarrhoea and piles. The gum is also useful in diarrhoea and dysentery. The transparent gummy substance oozing from the stem when cut or broken can be beneficially used in bowel affections. It also relieves tenesmus, that is, powerful straining to relieve the bowels.

Women's Disorders

A mixture of the ripe pulp of the fruit, cardamom, honey and cumin seeds, taken regularly in the morning tones up sagging breasts. It is also useful in preventing cancer of the breast and uterus and helps cure sterility due to a deficiency of the harmone progesterone. About 90 grams of the sap of the fresh bark, 2 corns of pepper, a few drops of pure cow's *ghee* and a dessertspoon of honey, prevents any post-partum complications. It is taken twice daily immediately after childbirth.

Children's Diseases

Juice of the tender leaves, given with milk and sugar, is very useful in bowel complaints of children. A powder of the leaves

175

can also be taken in 2 to 4 gram doses for the same complaints. The pulp of the ripe fruit can also be used beneficially in the treatment of stomach disorders of children. It should be given in 30 to 60 grams doses.

Urtecaria

About 30 ml of fresh leaf juice, mixed with cumin, is useful in the treatment of urtecaria--an allergic disease marked by painful red round weals on the skin. It should be taken twice daily.

Biliousness

The bark of the tree is good for biliousness. It can be taken either in the powdered or decoction form. The juice of the leaves can also be applied to the skin eruptions caused by biliousness.

Other Uses

Hiccups: Wood apple in the form of *chutney* or *sherbet* is useful in treating hiccups. It is made with salt and tamarind.

Aphrodisiac: Powder of the leaves, dried in shade, with an equal quantity of sugar candy is useful in spermatorrhoea, or involuntary ejaculation, premature ejaculation and functional impotency. One teaspoon of this powder is taken with cold water thrice daily in these disorders. About 20 grams of gum, dissolved in cow's milk and mixed with sugar, is also effective in spermatorrhoea and premature ejaculation. It can be taken thrice daily.

Part II

Ash Gourd

Botanical Name: *Benincasa hispida*
Indian Name: *Petha*

Description and Composition

Ash gourd, also known as white gourd or wax gourd, is an annual, hairy climbing herb. It is an ash-coloured, large fruit-vegetable like pumpkin. It is commonly cultivated for its nutritive and medicinal values.

An analysis of the ash gourd shows substantial amount of moisture and a little amount of protein, fat, fibre and carbohydrates. Its mineral and vitamin contents are calcium, phosphorus, iron, thiamine, riboflavin, niacin and vitamin C. Its calorific value is 15. The seeds contain a pale yellow oil.

Healing Power and Curative Properties

Ash gourd is wholesome and nutritive. Being low in calories it is particularly useful for diabetic and obese people. It is cooling and laxative. This herb increases the secretion and discharge of urine. It promotes libido and is useful in periodic attacks of hysteria and convulsions.

Peptic Ulcer

The dilute juice of ash gourd is beneficial in the treatment of peptic ulcer. The juice, squeezed out of grated ash gourd with an equal amount of water added to it, should be taken daily in the morning on an empty stomach. No food should be consumed for 2 to 3 hours afterwards. This also relieves inflammation in the alimentary canal.

Bleeding

Ash gourd acts as a blood coagulant. From ancient times, its fresh juice mixed with a teaspoon of *amla* or lime juice is used as a specific medicine to stop profuse bleeding from lungs and nose, in piles and haematuria, a disease characterised by the presence of blood cells in the urine.

General Debility

A delicious sweet prepared from pulp of the fruit by boiling its pieces in water and adding sugar syrup to it is used as a medicine to increase weight, in tuberculosis, weakness of the heart, heat in the body, thinness of semen and anaemia.

Intestinal Worms

Shelled seeds of ash gourd are anabolic —that promote tissue growth—especially when taken with coconut milk. They expel tape worm and other worms from the intestine.

Dandruff

The peel and seeds of ash gourd, boiled in coconut oil, are useful in hair growth, prevent dandruff and dryness of the scalp.

Other Uses

Detoxifying Effects: Due to its diuretic action, ash gourd increases the ouput of urine and washes out waste products from the body.

The unripe fruit is cooked as a vegetable. The ripe fruit is largely used for making sweetmeat. The young leaves and buds are also cooked.

Asoka

Botanical Name: *Saraca Indica*
Indian Name: *Ashoka*

Description and Composition

Asoka is a small, spreading, evergreen tree, with smooth brownish bark and compound leaves forming a dense crown. It has bright orange flowers in small dense branches and flat fruits with several smooth grey seeds. This tree has to be distinguished from the Indian fir or mast tree, botanically known as *polyalthia longifolia*. Asoka is one of the sacred trees of the Hindus.

The dried bark of the tree constitutes the drug. The bark contains tannins and catechol. B.N. Ghosh of the School of Tropical Medicine, Calcutta, investigated the powdered bark ash of Asoka and found presence of silica, sodium, potassium, phosphate, magnesium, iron, calcium, strontium and aluminium.[1] A crystalline glycosidal substance has been isolated from the bark, with galactose as the constituent sugar.

1. R.N. Chopra, I.C. Chopra, K.L. Handa and L.D. Kapur, Indigenous Drugs of India, 2nd edition reprint, p. 401-402, Academic Publishers, Calcutta, 1982.

Healing Power and Curative Properties

The bark is prescribed in Ayurvedic medicine for arresting bleeding or secretion and as a uterine sedative. It is said to have a stimulating effect on the endometrium that is, the mucuous membrane lining the uterus and on the ovarian tissues.

Uterine Disorders

The bark of the tree is effective for excessive blood loss during menstruation due to the presence of uterine fibroids, leucorrhoea and other causes. It can be used as a substitute for ergot, a kind of dried fungus used in medicine in the treatment of uterine hamorrhages. It is taken as a decoction.

About 90 grams of the bark is boiled in 30 ml of milk and 360 ml of water till the total quantity is reduced to about 90 grams. This is divided in 2 or 3 doses to be given in a day. The treatment should commence from the fourth day of the menstruation and continue till the bleeding is checked. Fresh decoction is to be made every day.

Piles

The bark is also effective for internal piles. A decoction prepared in the same manner as in case of uterine disorders is taken in this condition.

Dysentery

The decoction is also useful in dysentery. A fluid extract of the flowers can be taken with beneficial results in haemorrhagic dysentery. This extract is prepared by grinding the flowers with water. It is taken in doses of 15 to 60 drops.

Other Diseases

The dried flowers of Asoka tree are useful in diabetes. The bark of the tree is also useful in treating scorpion-sting.

Bay Berry

Botanical Name: *Myrica nagi*
Indian Name: *Kaiphala*

Description and Composition

Bay berry is an aromatic tree growing upto 10 metres high. The leaves of the tree are 7.5 cms long, pale to rust coloured and alternate. The tree has hairy stalks with minute flowers growing solitary or on a common drooping stalk. It has wrinkled seeds.

The herb contains tannins, triterpenes (including myricadiol), flavonoid glycosides, resin and gum.

Healing Power and Curative Properties

The bark of the tree is aromatic, stimulant, tonic and resolvent. It is useful in arresting secretion or bleeding and in expelling wind from the stomach. It is also an antiseptic. Myricitrin in bay berry is bactericidal and encourages the flow of bile. Another constituent of the herb, myricadiol is reported to cause retention of salt and excretion of potassium.

Fevers and Colds

Bay berry is a valuable remedy in fevers and colds. A hot decoction of the herb can be taken in the treatment of fevers, catarrh of the mucous membranes, affections of the chest and typhoid. The powdered bark can be used as a snuff for congested nasal passages, which are relieved by sneezing. The decoction also makes a good gargle for throat infections.

Intestinal Disorders

Bay berry is also used to treat inflammation and infection of the gastro-intestinal tract.

Women's Diseases

The herb taken internally can be used to treat post-partum haemorrhage. It can also be used as a douche for excessive menstrual bleeding and leucorrhoea, or white discharge.

Respiratory Disorders

Bay berry is highly beneficial in treating respiratory disorders like asthma and chronic bronchitis. Its bark may be taken either in a decoction or powdered form, as in the case of fevers and colds.

Teeth Disorders

A paste of the bark made with vinegar can be used for strengthening gums and relieving toothache.

Wounds and Ulcers

A compress of the herb can be used for dressing wounds and ulcers. The powder of its bark can be dusted over putrid sores.

Other Diseases

Bay berry is useful in several other diseases like diarrhoea, dysentery and chronic gonorrhoea. A decoction of the herb can be taken with cinnamon in chronic cough and piles.

Bitter Chamomile

Botanical Name: *Matricaria chamomilla*
Indian Name: *Babunah or Babuni-ke-phul*

Description and Composition

Bitter chamomile, also known as German chamomile, is an erect, aromatic, annual herb with several branches growing upto 20 to 45 cms high. It has thread-like leaves. Terminal flower-heads are about 2.5 cm across, on slender branched stalks, bearing an outer whorl of 10 to 20 white flowers with a yellow centre. The flowers of the plant constitute the drug chamomile.

The herb contains a volatile oil. This oil consists of chamazulene, farnesene and bisabolol. Other constituents of chamomile are flavonoids, coumarins, plant acids, fatty acids, cyanogenic glycosides salicylate derivatives, polysaccharides, choline, amino acids and tannin.

Healing Power and Curative Properties

Bitter chamomile flowers contain many medicinal virtues. They relieve flatulence, induce copious perspiration and regulate menstrual periods.They are also stimulant and useful in dissolving or absorbing a tumour or any coagulated fluids in the body.

183

Digestive Disorders

Chamomile is an effective remedy for digestive disorders, specially of nervous origin. It can be used beneficially in dyspepsia, flatulence and colic. A powder of the flowers or 1 to 3 drops of oil extracted from flowers is taken in 1 to 2 gram doses in the treatment of such disorders. A cold infusion of the flowers is useful in indigestion and summer diarrhoea in doses of 30 to 60 grams.

Insomnia

Chamomile is useful in insomnia. An infusion of its flowers induces sleep.

Women's Diseases

A warm infusion of the flowers is taken in the treatment of painful and difficult menstruation.

Children's Problems

An infusion of the flowers has a relaxing effect and is of special value to hyperactive children. It acts as a nervine sedative and tonic on the gastro-intestinal canal. The flowers are useful for earache, neuralgic pains, stomach disorders, convulsions and ailments caused by dentition.

Skin Diseases

Two of the components, bisabolol and chamazulene contained in the volatile oil of the herb are powerful antiseptics. Chamazulene relieves pain, promotes healing of wounds and is anti-inflammatory and anti-spasmodic. Applied externally, it helps recovery from burns and soothes eczema. Recent investigations show that bisabolol speeds up healing of ulcers and prevents reoccurrence.

Rheumatism

Chamomile is also useful in treating rheumatic afflictions, where its extracted oil, diluted in a vegetable oil is, rubbed on the affected parts. It eases the pain of rheumatism and gout. A compress of chamomile flowers is used to treat sciatica.

Bloodwort

Botanical Name: *Achillea millefolium*
Indian Name: *Rojmari or Gandana*

Description and Composition

Bloodwort is an erect herb, 30 to 60 cms high, with fine soft, hair. It has leafy, grooved stems and alternate, oblong tapering leaves, 5 to 10 cms long. Its flowers are small and crowded with thin scales. The fruits are flat, oblong shaped and shining.

The herb contains volatile oil, lactones, flavonoids, tannins, coumarins, saponins, sterols, a bitter glyco alkaloid, cyanidin, aminoacids and acid sugars.

Healing Power and Curative Properties

Bloodwort is bitter, aromatic, stimulant and tonic. It is useful in arresting bleeding. It induces copious perspiration.

Fevers

Bloodwort is one of the best known herbal remedies for fevers. A hot infusion of the herb induces perspiration which cools fevers and expels toxins.

High Blood Pressure

The herb is useful in treating high blood pressure. Like all sweat-inducing remedies, bloodwort encourages blood flow to the skin which helps lower blood pressure. It is the alkaloid in bloodwort which has been reported to lower blood pressure.

Stomach Disorders

Bloodwort is a valuable remedy for several stomach disorders like colic, heartburn and flatulence. About 30 grams of its decoction may be taken every hour in the treatment of these disorders. A dessertspoon of fresh juice of the herb, taken thrice a day, aids digestion and gastric disorders.

Piles

As it arrests bleeding, a decoction or infusion of the herb is useful in bleeding piles. The powdered leaves and flower-heads are useful as carminative to relieve flatulence when given in 6 to 30 centigram doses.

Women's Disorders

A hot infusion of the leaves is a powerful emmenagogue (a drug which induces menses) and thus useful in promoting and regulating menstrual cycles. In case of irregular menstrual flow, about 30 grams of decoction of the herb can be taken every hour with beneficial results. The essential oil extracted from its flowers has proved beneficial in the treatment of disorders of the female reproductive organs. About 5 to 30 drops of the oil can be taken in treating such disorders.

Wounds

Bloodwort is an effective wound healer. The tannins in it are probably responsible for this property. It is good for all kinds of bleeding, both external and internal.

Calamus

Botanical Name: *Acorus calamus*
Indian Name: *Bach*

Description and Composition

Calamus, also known as sweet-flag, is a perennial herb with long creeping and aromatic rhizomes or underground stems sprouting leaves. The flowering shoots of the plant are supported by a large leaf-like structure called spathe. It has pale-green, small flowers, in 5 to 10 cm long cylindric spikes and yellowish fruits. The dried rhizomes of the plant constitute the drug calamus and is used in medicine.

The dry rhizomes of calamus contain a yellow aromatic oil. The essential oil contains calamen, calamenos, calameon and asarone. Indian calameon oil contains asarone, small amounts of sesquiterpenes and sesquiterpene alcohols. The odour of the oil is ascribed to an unidentified constituent. The leaves contain oxalic acid and calcium.

Healing Power and Curative Properties

The rhizomes are of great medicinal value.The root-stock of the plant is an aromatic stimulant, bitter tonic and expectorant. It relieves flatulence, counteracts spasmodic disorders and induces vomiting. It regulates menstural periods. It is also laxative, diuretic and aphrodisiac.

Stomach Disorders

Calamus gives relief to heavy stomach by relieving flatulence, colic and increasing appetite. The burnt root mixed with some bland oil such as refined coconut oil or a poultice of the root may be applied over the abdomen in treatment.

Diarrhoea and Dysentery

The drug is a time-tested remedy and is an ingredient in Ayurvedic medicines for chronic diarrhoea. It is also effective in chronic dysentery, due to the presence of tannins. Its infusion can be given to children suffering from these ailments.

Asthma

Calamus is highly beneficial in the treatment of asthma; it removes catarrhal matter and phlegm from the bronchial tubes. About 65 centigrams of the herb is taken every 2 or 3 hours in this condition.

Common Cold

The herb is also useful in treating common cold. A small piece of the rhizome is roasted and powdered. A pinch of this powder taken with honey provides great relief. For infants, the paste of calamus mixed in breast milk is touched on the baby's tongue. Another convenient method of giving the medicine to infants is to apply a little paste on the mother's nipples.

Whooping Cough

The powder of the roasted herb is an effective home remedy for children suffering from whooping cough. A pinch of this powder can be given with honey. Being antispasmodic, it prevents the severe bouts of coughing. For smaller children, the dose must be proportionately smaller.

Intestinal Worms

Calamus is effective in expelling intestinal worms. The powdered root is taken for this purpose.

Mouth Disorders

The herb is useful in treating mouth ulcers, coating on tongue and rawness, that is, inflammation of the skin. A small piece of the herb should be rubbed on the tongue to obtain relief.

Chalmogra

Botanical Name: *Hydnocarpus laurifolia*
Indian Name: *Garudphal*

Description and Composition

Chalmogra is a tall evergreen tree with whitish wood. It has sharply-toothed, smooth and shining leaves, spherical fruits, about the size of an apple, with a rough thick brown rind. Within the fruit there are 10 to 20 angular seeds, embedded in a scanty white pulp. The trade name chalmogra is based on the local name of the tree.

Chalmogra has been used in the Ayurvedic system of medicine for leprosy since many centuries. In ancient Buddhist literature the efficacy of raw chalmogra seeds in treating leprosy is mentioned. Records show that the oil extracted from its seeds has been used in the treatment of leprosy and other skin diseases since 1595. In the *Makhzanel-Adwiya*, one of the oldest books on Mohammedan materia medica, mention is made of the use of the seeds under the name of chalmogri.

By 1868, the curative effects of chalmogra were so well-known that it was made official in the Pharmacopoeia of India. It was, however, not till 1904, when Fredrick B. Power and his collaborators published in detail the chemistry of chalmogra oil, that the attention of the scientific world was drawn to this valuable drug. Experiments have proven its bactricidal properties.

The seeds of chalmogra yield a fatty oil. The oil contains hydnocarpic acid, oleic acid and palmitic acid

Healing Power and Curative Properties

The oil from the seeds has medicinal properties. It is a tonic, useful in correcting disordered processes of nutrition and in restoring the normal function of the system. It is also a local stimulant.

Fevers

The bark of the tree contains tannins, which are beneficial in the treatment of fevers.

Leprosy

The oil extracted from the seeds is useful in leprosy. It should be applied locally to the affected parts. Recently chalmogra has been recognised in the allopathic medicine as a valuable remedy for leprosy.

Skin Disorders

Chalmogra oil is a specific medicine for treating skin diseases. It is locally used in rheumatism and phthisis or tuberculosis. It is an effective dressing for scaly eruptions and chronic skin diseases, even those of syphilitic origin. A liniment made of equal parts of the oil and lime water is applied to scald heads, leprous ulcerations, rheumatic pains and scruf, or a scaly condition, on the head.

A paste of the seeds is a domestic remedy for wounds and certain skin diseases like eczema, ringworm and scabies. The infusion is used as a disinfectant for vaginal infection in gonorrhoea and foetid discharges, especially after childbirth.

Chirayata

Botanical Name: *Swertia chirata*
Indian Name: *Chirayata*

Description and Composition

Chirayata, also known as Indian gentian is a robust annual herb which grows upto about 1.5 meters in height. It has leaves in opposite pairs about 10 cms long, without stalks, pointed at the tip. The plant has numerous flowers, pale green in colour, tinged with purple, with long white or pink hairs and minute sharp pointed fruits. The whole plant, collected in its flowering stage and dried, constitutes the drug. The trade name chirayata is based on the local name of the plant. It has long been used by the Aurvedic physicians as a bitter tonic.

The plant contains a bitter glycoside chiratin, which yields on hydrolysis, two bitter principles, ophelic acid and chiratin. The latter is soluble in water. The ophelic acid is a brown hydroscopic substance which is soluble in water and alcohol. It also contains resin, tannin and 4 to 8 per cent of ash.

Healing Power and Curative Properties

Chirayata is a valuable bitter tonic. It is laxative and an appetizer. It also corrects the disordered process of nutrition and restores the normal function of the system.

Fevers

Chirayata is an effective drug for reducing fevers. It is specially beneficial in the treatment of malarial fevers. It is also effective in hysteria and convulsions.

Stomach Disorders

The herb is an excellent drug for strengthening the stomach and promoting its action. It is used in the treatment of dyspepsia and diarrhoea.

Intestinal Worms

Chirayata possesses anthelmintic, that is, worms destroying, properties and is used in killing intestinal worms. An infusion of the herb is taken for this purpose.

General Debility

It serves as an effective tonic in case of general weakness and during convalescence. The infusion of the plant can be taken in doses of 60 ml or 4 tablespoons twice a day, before meals.

Preparation and Doses: The herb is used in the form of an infusion or tincture. The infusion is prepared in hot water with aromatics like cloves and cinnamon. It is generally taken in doses of 15 to 30 ml or 1 to 2 tablespoons.

Other Uses

Hiccups: The root of the plant is useful in checking hiccups and vomiting. It is taken in doses of 0.5 to 2 grams with honey.

Colchicum

Botanical Name: *Colchicum luteum*
Indian Name: *Hirantutiya*

Description and Composition

Colchicum is an annual herb with brownish fleshy underground stems. It is almost conical in shape, flattened on one side and round on the other. The plant has very narrow leaves, broadening towards the tip, large yellow flowers and fruits with recurved tips.

190

The chief constituent of colchicum is the alkaloid, colchicine, which occurs in the form of yellow flakes, crystals or as whitish yellow amorphous powder. Its odour resembles the hay when dampened and warmed.

Healing Power and Curative Properties

It is a medicine of great repute in Afghanistan and northern India. The medicinal properties were well known even amongst the Arabs. Its corms and seeds are incorporated in the British Pharmacopoeia and allopathic medicine alludes it as a remedy for gout.

Gout

The active principle colchicine contained in the corms is useful in relieving pain and inflammations of gout. Clinical experiments with colchicum in small doses over a long period have shown success in about 60 per cent of patients. The seeds, chiefly the rind also contain colchicine, and may be used in the treatment of gout in the same manner as the corms.

Rheumatism

The drug is beneficial in the treatment of rheumatic swelling. A paste made with saffron and egg can be applied beneficially to rheumatic and other swellings.

Wounds

Dried and powdered root of the plant is useful in the healing of wounds. It should be sprinkled on the affected area.

Precautions: It has a very bitter taste, and darkens on exposure to light. It has similar action as colchicine, but the latter is more active and toxic. When taken in large doses, colchinine causes intestinal pain, diarrhoea and vomiting. The use of the drug can cause severe irritation in the intestines. To counteract this, it is advisable to use the drug with belladonna or hyoscyamus *(khurasana ajwain)*.

Devil's Tree

Botanical Name: *Alstonia scholaris*
Indian Name: *Saitan-ka-jhad, Chhatim*

Description and Composition

Devil's tree is a large evergreen tree about 25 metres high. It has a bitter milky juice, rough, dark grey bark and whorled branches. Its leaves are small and it has greenish-white flowers. Its fruits are long, narrow and slender. The dried bark of the tree constitutes the drug.

The bark of the tree contains many alkaloids. Of these, the most important are ditamine and ditain. The latter is an uncrystallisable bitter principle to which are ascribed the febrifuge, that is, the thirst quenching properties of the drug.

Healing Power and Curative Properties

The bark of the devil's tree has been reputed in the indigenious system of medicines for ages as a tonic and a drug which restores the normal function of the digestive system. It is also useful in fevers and skin diseases.

Fevers

The herb is an excellent substitute for cinchona and quinine for the treatment of intermittent and remittent fevers. Its powder can be taken in doses of 2 to 6 grams or its extract should be given in doses of 2 to 10 drops.

An infusion of the bark is very useful in malaria. It brings down fever steadily to normal in a short time without causing perspiration and over exhaustion which usually follows other medicines for malaria.

Bowel Complaints

Chhatim is effective in bowel complaints. About 33 centigrams of the powder of the bark can be given in these complaints.

Catarrhal Dyspepsia

The powdered bark is beneficial in the treatment of catarrhal dyspepsia—that is indigestion accompanied by discharge of mucus from the inflamed mucous membrane of the intestines. About 3.25 grams of the powder can be given at night.

Diarrhoea and Dysentery

The drug is an effective remedy in chronic diarrhoea and in advanced stage of dysentery. It, however, does not seem to produce any marked effect in ordinary diarrhoea.

Skin Disorders

For skin diseases such as eczema, acne and ringworm, an infusion of the bark is given in 30 to 60 ml doses, twice or thrice a day.

Digitalis

Botanical Name: *Digitalis.purpurea*
Indian Name: *Tilpushpi*

Description and Composition

Digitalis, commonly known as Foxglove, is a biennial or perennial herb growing upto about 1.2 metres tall. The lower basal leaves of the plant are long-stalked, hairy and egg-shaped and the upper leaves are almost without stalks, becoming smaller in size as they go upwards. It has white or purple flowers, and egg-shaped fruits.

The active constituents of digitalis are the several glycosides, including three well defined glycosides, namely, digitoxin, gitoxin and gitalin. All the three glycosides possess the property to promote and stimulate cardio-vascular activity. Leaves contain little amount of glycosides. Digitoxin is also contained in the leaves. Its seeds contain an amber coloured fatty oil with bland taste.

Healing Power and Curative Properties

The tinctures from the Indian leaves are darker and contain more resinous matter than those prepared from the European varieties.

Heart Disorders

This drug is mainly used in treating heart diseases. In case of congested heart failure, it promotes and stimulates the activity of all muscle tissues. The herb forces more blood into the coronaries thereby improving the nourishment to the heart.

When blood circulation gets impaired and dropsy sets in, digitalis helps in restoration and regulation of the function of the heart.

Kidney Disorders

It helps urination by improving the blood supply to the kidneys and removes obstructions within the kidneys.

Wounds and Burns

Digitalis is used in some ointments for local application on wounds and burns. In cases of burns, it is very effective in preserving severely damaged cells.

Methods for Uses and Dosages: Digitalis is commonly administered in the form of tablets, powder or digitalis tincture and suppositories available with the Ayurvedic pharmacies. It is also used in making injections. In therapeutic doses, the drug usually produces mild toxic effects. The toxic effects include headache, fatigue, drowsiness, nausea, vomiting and blurred vision. It is therefore, necessary to regulate the dose in such a manner so as to avoid such effects. The toxic effects mentioned should be watched carefully and the dose regulated accordingly.

East Indian Rosebay

Botanical Name: *Ervatamia coronaria*
Indian Name: *Chandi or taggar*

Description and Composition

East Indian Rosebay is a small perennial shrub. It has a round stem of about 25 cms diameter, with a greyish white, rough, cracked, silvery bark. It grows upto two metres in height.

The plant has numerous branches forming a dense crown. It has long, simple, elliptic leaves, dark green in colour. The flowers are large, soft white and very delicate with a sweet fragrance. The plant produces a thick milky juice when any part is cut.

East Indian Rosebay contains alkaloids, tabernaemontanine and coronarine, a crystalline resin alcohol, caoutchouc and some other substances.

Healing Power and Curative Properties

The leaves of the plant do not have any prominent taste. When crushed, they turn soapy. The cellulose content is very soft. It is used in curing worms and certain skin disorders.

Intestinal Worms

The root of the plant is anthelmintic and is used for killing intestinal worms. The milky juice of the plant too has similar property and is used for this purpose.

Toothache

For allaying toothache, the root of the plant is chewed.

Eye Disorders

The herb is beneficial in the treatment of several eye disorders. A paste of the plant made with water and lime juice or the latex of the plant mixed with lime juice can be applied to clear opacity of the cornea of the eyes. The juice or the milk from the leaves, either by themselves or mixed with charcoal of the plant, can be used with beneficial results as a soothing application in opthalmia, that is, inflammation of the eye.

The juice of the flowers mixed with some bland oil such as refined coconut oil can be used with gratifying results for sore eyes and inflammation of the cornea.

Skin Disorders

East Indian rosebay is valuable in certain skin disorders. The juice of the leaves is a soothing application in skin irritation and wounds. The herb is useful as a local anodyne and relieves pain. The latex mixed with the juice makes a soothing dressing for wounds. It also prevents inflammations.

Preparation and Doses: About 20 grams of the leaves of East Indian rosebay plant with five grams of holy basil (*tulsi*) or ecliplta alba (*bringaraj*) may be chewed well and swallowed. Fresh petals can also be used with the leaves.

Euphorbia

Botanical Name: *Euphorbia hirta*
Indian Name: *Lal dudhi*

Description and Composition

Euphorbia is an annual herb, ascending or erect upto 50 cms high. It grows as a weed and is known by various names like Australian asthma weed, snake weed and cat's hair. It has round stems, covered with yellowish hairs, small leaves, dark green on the upper side and pale on the lower side and minute whitish flowers in small stalked clusters. It has small hairy fruits; and 3-angled, wrinkled, light reddish brown seeds. The entire plant, collected in flowering and fruit bearing stages and dried, constitutes the drug.

The herb attracted the attention of allopathic physicians many years ago. They came to India and it was at their instance that the drug was introduced into Europe somewhere around 1884. The alcoholic extract of the whole plant is used in modern allopathic medicine.

The chemistry of the drug shows it to contain gallic acid, quercetin, a new phenolic substance, traces of an essential oil besides those of an alkaloid.

Healing Power and Curative Properties

The leaves are useful in arresting bleeding and in counteracting spasmodic disorders. They relieve feverishness and produce a feeling of coolness. They have a soothing effect on the skin and the mucous membranes. They serve as a mild laxative. Leaves have a hard cellulose content. Raw juice, paste, powder and decoction can be made from 15 grams of these leaves and mixed with 5 grams of holy basil or *tulsi*.

Respiratory Disorders

The drug enjoys a great reputation in Ayurvedic system of medicine and is believed to be a most effective remedy for diseases of the respiratory tract in general, especially cough, coryza or colds in the head, bronchitis and asthma. It has a depressant action on the heart and respiration besides producing a relaxation of the bronchioles.

Diarrhoea

Euphorbia is useful in treating diarrhoea. About 12 grams of the herb ground in water can be taken to check the disease.

Genito-Urinary Disorders

Euphorbia is beneficial in the treatment of gonorrhoea and other venereal diseases. The plant is also useful in impotency, premature ejacueation and spermatorrhoea or involuntary ejaculation.

Intestinal Worms

Its leaves possess anthelmintic properties and are useful in treating intestinal worms amongst children.

Problem of Breast Milk Secretion

The plant is very helpful in promoting formation and flow of breast milk amongst nursing mothers.

Skin Disorders

The leaves of the plant are useful in the treatment of skin disorders like ulcers. The paste of the plant can also be applied beneficially on wounds and burns. The milky juice of the plant is useful in the treatment of warts. It should be applied externally on the affected area.

Cracked Lips and Tongue

The milky juice of the plant can be applied on lips and tongue, in case of cracking or chapping.

Precautions: The drug should not be taken in large doses as it may cause irritation in the stomach and result in vomiting.

Other Uses

Hair Tonic: Applied on the head, the milky juice of the plant is useful in promoting hair growth.

Fennel

Botanical Name: *Fenniculum vulgare*
Indian Name: *Saunf*

Description and Composition

Fennel is a yellewish green, biennial or perennial herb commonly cultivated throughout India. It has been used for flavouring from ancient times. The whole plant is aromatic.

An analysis of fennel shows it to consist of moisture 6.3 per cent, protein 9.5 per cent, fat 10 per cent, minerals 13.4 per cent, fibre 18.5 per cent and carbohydrates 42.3 per cent. Its mineral and vitamin contents are calcium, phosphorus, iron, sodium, potassium, thiamine, riboflavin, niacin and vitamin C. Its calorific value is 370.

The composition of the oil varies widely according to the variety and origin. Indian fennel oil contains substantial amount of anethole and fenchone. It possesses a sweet taste. The fatty acids of the oil are palmitic acid and petroselinic acid.

Healing Power and Curative Properties

The leaves of fennel are digestive, appetizing and stimulating. They increase the secretion and discharge of urine. The seeds are sweet, laxative, aphrodisiac and arrest bleeding. They also relieve flatulence and promote the removal of catarrhal matter and phlegm from the bronchial tubes. Oil of fennel, distilled from the dry seeds is aromatic, carminative and antispasmodic. It is used in various carminative preparations.

Digestive Disorders

The use of fennel is well known as a digetive aid. It may be given in small quantities to help young children digest carbohydrates. An infusion prepared by boiling a tablespoon of fennel seeds in 100 ml of water for half an hour, is highly beneficial in indigestion, biliousness, flatulence, constipation and atonic dyspepsia. Chewing its seeds after meals prevent foul breath, indigestion, constipation and vomiting.

Colic

Fennel is one of the safest herbs for colic, for helping the baby to release gas and relieve tummy. It may be used in combination with other herbs like peppermint and crushed caraway seeds or alone. A teaspoon of the herbs is boiled in a cup of water, and allowed to steep in the water for about 20 minutes. This is strained and allowed to cool. This tea, given to the baby in his feed bottle, helps cure colic. Not more than a teaspoon or two should be given at a time.

Respiratory Disorders

Leaves of fennel are useful in respiratory disorders like asthma and bronchitis. The juice may be given in the treatment of such conditions. Eating fennel seeds with figs is also a good medicine for cough, bronchitis and lung abscesses.

Menstrual Disorders

Fennel seeds promote menstruation and regulate monthly periods. An infusion of the seeds can be given in painful menstruation and other menstrual irregularities.

Eye Disorders

It is believed that fennel benefits the eyes. Herbalists today recommend bathing the weakened, sore or inflamed eyes with fennel tea. Regular application of the leaf-juice boiled with honey, is said to cure conjuctivitis.

Gokulakanta

Botanical Name: *Asteracantha longifolia or Hygrophila spinosa*
Indian Name: *Gokhulakanta*

Description and Composition

Gokulakanta is a stout, rough, thorny, slightly tall annual herb. The stem of the plant is thin and small, round, hairy and red in colour. The plant grows vertically upto about one metre with no branches on the sides. The leaves are simple, with waving or curling margins and the flowers are bright blue in colour. The seeds are small, flat, round, dark red in colour. The whole plant is covered with a soft hair growth. The entire plant is used medicinally, specially its leaves and roots.

The roots of the plant contain an essential oil. Its seeds contain a yellow semi-drying oil—that is, the oil which possesses the property to dry partially by evaporation. They also contain

diastase, lipase and protease. An alkaloid is also present in the
ds in addition to these chemical substances.

Healing Power and Curative Properties

The herb is a tonic and stimulant. It increases the secretion
and discharge of urine and promotes libido. The ash of the plant
serves as an excellent diuretic. It has a soothing effect on the skin
and mucous membranes.

Dropsy

The ash of the plant is useful in treating dropsy, a disease
marked by an excessive collection of watery fluids in the tissues
or cavities of the body. The ash should be administered
preferably with cow's urine in doses of 1.5 to 3 grams. The root
is also useful for treating dropsy.

Genito-Urinary Disorders

The root of the plant is beneficial in the treatment of
gonorrhoea and urinary disorders, including inflammation of the
urinary tract and stone in the kidneys. Its decoction can be given
in doses of 30 to 60 grams, twice or thrice a day.

The decoction of its leaves can be used with confidence in
case of syphilis and gonorrhoea. The mucilage obtained by
infusing the seeds in water is also prescribed in gonorrhoea,
urinary diseases and as a tonic.

Liver Disorders

The root of the plant is useful in treating liver disorders like
jaundice and hepatitis. It is specially useful in hepatic
derangement. A decoction of the root is administered in the
treatment of such conditions. About 60 grams of the root is
boiled in half a litre of water for 20 to 30 minutes in a closed
vessel. About 30 to 60 ml of this preparation is given two or
three time daily.

Anaemia

The herb purifies blood and is beneficial in the treatment
of anaemia. A decoction of its root can be administered in the
same manner as for liver disorders.

Rheumatism

The drug is also effective in rheumatic afflictions such as
rheumatism, arthritis, and gout.

Methods for Uses and Dosages: The leaves of the plant do not have any noticeable taste. They contain a cellulose which is hard. The leaves can be taken by themselves or mixed with the leaves of holy basil (*tulsi*). The juice from 20 grams of leaves can be mixed with either buttermilk or coconut water or fruit juice. Two teaspoons of the powdered leaves can also be mixed with 120 to 180 ml of buttermilk or 100 ml of water.

Hermal

Botanical Name: *Peganum harmala*
Indian Name: *Hermal*

Description and Composition
Hermal, also known as wild rue or Syrian rue, is a bushy herb with leaves divided into numerous narrow segments. It has white solitary flowers, capsular, spherical fruits and brownish seeds in various shapes. The dried seeds of the plant constitute the drug. The trade name is based on the local Indian name of the herb.

The seeds contain four alkaloids, harmine, harmaline, harmolol and peganine. The blossoms and stems yield alkaloid peganine identified with l'-peganine.

Healing Power and Curative Properties
The drug stimulates motor tracts of cerebrum and the central nervous system. In indigenous medicine, the herb is considered useful in restoring the disordered nutrition process besides as a purifier and aphrodisiac. Experiments have confirmed the bactericidal action of the drug.

Fevers
Hermal is beneficial in the treatment of remittent and intermittent fevers. It is useful in chronic malaria but is not so effective in acute cases. The seeds are given either as an infusion, decoction or in powder form.

Asthma
The drug is useful in asthma. The powder of the seeds given in doses of 2 to 8 grams, provides relief.

Tapeworm

Hermal seeds are effective in treating tapeworm infestation. The alkaloid hermaline has been found to have anthelmintic action. The powder of its seeds should be given for expelling worms. The herb as such has narcotic properties and can be used to induce deep sleep in cases of insomnia.

Menstrual Disorders

The herb is beneficial in painful and difficult menstruation and for regulating the menstrual periods. A decoction of the seeds is given in 15 to 30 ml doses.

Problem of Breast Milk Secretion

Hermal seeds are gatactogogue, that is, an agent which stimulates the secretion of breast milk or increases milk flow in nursing mothers.

Laryngitis

The drug is beneficial in the treatment of laryngitis, that is, inflammation of the larynx. A decoction of the seeds is used as a mouthwash.

Head Lice

Hermal is useful in killing head lice. A paste of the roots made with mustard oil should be applied externally.

Precautions: The drug should be used only in the prescribed doses. In higher doses, it may prove poisonous and bring about severe depressant action on the nervous system.

Hyssop

Botanical Name: *Hyssopus officinalis*
Indian Name: *Zufah yabis*

Description and Composition

Hyssop is a smooth, aromatic, perennial herb, 30 to 60 cms high. It has erect or diffused branches; linear oblong, lance-shaped leaves with a blunt or rounded apex and bluish purple flowers. Hyssop comes from the Hebrew name Esob. Hippocrates, the father of medicine, prescribed hyssop for chest complaints.

Hyssop contains volatile oil, fat, sugar, choline, tannins, carotene and xanthophyll. The tops contains ursolic acid. A glucoside diosmin which, on hydrolysis yields rhamnose, glucose and the aglucone diosmetin, have also been isolated.

Healing Power and Curative Properties

Hyssop is a stimulant and a tonic. It increases the secretion and discharge of urine and removes any obstruction to body secretion or excretion by opening the natural passages or pores of the body. It also induces movement of the bowels.

Respiratory Disorders

Herbalists recommend hyssop for treating a wide range of respiratory disorders such as influenza, colds, catarrh and bronchitis. Marrubiin, a bitter principle in the plant, has expectorant qualities and helps to promote the removal of catarrhal matter and phlegm from the bronchial tubes. Hyssop extracts have exhibited antiviral activities, especially against the herpes simplex virus that causes cold sores. An infusion or a syrup of its leaves can be taken in coughs, asthma, sore throat and chronic bronchitis with beneficial results.

Roundworms

Hyssop is useful in killing intestinal worms. An infusion of the herb or juice of the leaves taken twice or thrice daily expells roundworms.

Digestive Disorders

Hyssop is useful in digestive disorders. It strengthens the stomach and promotes its action. It can be given beneficially with honey in dyspepsia and flatulence.

Skin Disorders

A paste of the herb applied externally to the affected parts is an effective remedy for skin conditions like bruises, wounds and burns. It is also good for blackeye, sprains and strains. The paste steeped in boiling water can be used to foment contused wounds, black eye, sprains and strains.

Other Diseases

The herb is also useful in uterine and urinary disorders. The infusion of the herb is a useful gargle for sore throat and a wash for sore eyes.

Indian Acalypha

Botanical Name: *Acalypha indica*
Indian Name: *Khokali or Kuppi*

Description and Composition

Indian acalypha is an erect annual herb, growing upto 75 cms. It has numerous long, angular, branches covered with soft hair. Its thin egg-shaped leaves have a smooth surface. The flowers are in erect, long spikes. It has small hairy fruits; and minute pale brown seeds. The whole plant is collected in its flowering stage and dried.

The plant contains the alkaloid acalyphine which is an active principle.

Healing Power and Curative Properties

The roots, leaves and young shoots of the plant have medicinal value. The drug increases the secretion and discharge of urine and is a laxative. The juice of the leaves is an efficient emetic for inducing vomiting. The root in small doses is expectorant and nauseant. It helps remove catarrhal matter and phlegm from the bronchial tubes.

Croup

The herb is of special value in treating croup, a disease mostly occuring in children. It is characterised by cough and difficulty in breathing and is caused by an obstruction in the larynx. The herb is safe to use in this condition and also acts fast. The juice can be administered in doses of 1 teaspoon. The dose may be increased to 4 teaspoons according to age.

Intestinal Worms

The herb is useful in killing intestinal worms. The juice of the leaves or their decoction, mixed with a little garlic, can be given for such symptoms.

Constipation

A decoction of the leaves is an effective laxative and thus is useful in constipation. A suppository of the fresh leaves, introduced in the rectum of small children suffering from constipation, induces free motions.

Skin Diseases

The drug is useful as an external application in skin diseases. A paste of its fresh leaves is applied to the affected parts. The juice of fresh leaves can be applied for scabies and other skin diseases, such as syphilitic ulcers, bedsores, maggot-infested sores and wounds.

Rheumatism

Indian acalypha is a popular remedy in rheumatism. The juice of the fresh leaves is applied mixed with lime and onion. A mixture of the fresh juice and oil can be applied in rheumatic arthritis.

Indian Aloe

Botanical Name: *Aloe barbadensis*
Indian Name: *Ghee kanvar or Musabbar*

Description and Composition

Indian aloe is an erect plant, 30 to 150 cm in height. It has smooth, pale green, fleshy leaves, convex below, tapering to a blunt point, with horny prickles at the margins. It has yellow or orange coloured cylindrical flowers. The bitter juice of the fleshy leaves is used in medicine.

The active principle of aloe is a mixture of glycosides called aloin. The proportion of aloin varies in different specimens of aloes. The chief constituent of aloin is barbaloin which is a pale-yellow crystalline glycoside, soluble in water. The other constituents include isobarbaloin, aloe-emodin (a hydrolytic product of barbaloin), resins and some water soluble substance. The characteristic odour is due to traces of an essential oil.

Healing Power and Curative Properties

The leaves of the plant possess many medicinal properties. They are useful in restoring the disordered processes of nutrition. They promote libido and arrest secretion or bleeding. They also promote and regulate the menstrual periods.

Liver Disorders

The herb stimulates the liver and is useful in liver and

spleen disorders. It can be used in jaundice and enlargement of liver, spleen and other glands. The pulp of one leaf should be administered with black salt and ginger every morning for 10 days in the treatment of such disorders.

Colds
The drug is valuable in colds and coughs. The juice of the roasted leaf should be taken with honey for treatment.

Rheumatism
Indian aloe is useful in lumbago, sciatica and rheumatism. The pulp of one leaf is taken daily for relief.

Indigestion
The herb is useful in stomach disorders. The leaves strengthen the functioning of stomach and promote its action. A salad of its leaves is beneficial in cases of indigestion, constipation and flatulence.

Intestinal Worms
The leaves have the property to kill intestinal worms in children. The condensed leaf juice, after boiling the leaves in water, is a popular and effective home remedy.

Skin Disorders
The use of the herb in treating inflamed and painful parts of the body is common in Indian medicine. The fresh juice from its leaves should be applied externally.

Indian Barberry

Botanical Name: *Berberris aristata*
Indian Name: *Rasaut*

Description and Composition
Indian Barberry is a large thorny shrub with yellow wood and whitish or pale grey branches. The dried roots of the plant constitute the drug. The chief constituent of the drug is berberine, a bitter alkaloid. Two alkaloid chlorides, namely palmatine chloride and a mixture of palmatine and berberine chlorides have also been isolated from the plant.

Healing Power and Curative Properties

Indian barberry has been made official in the Pharmacopoeia of India. Mohideen Sheriff, a well-known authority on herbs considers it an important indigenous medicine and brought it to the notice of the medical profession.[1]

The herb is useful in restoring the disordered processes of nutrition and restores the normal function of the system. It helps open the natural ducts or pores of the body, arrests bleeding and induces copious perspiration despite its astringent properties. Anti-tubercular activity has also been attributed to this drug.

Fevers

Indian barberry is as valuable as quinine in malarial fevers. It is particularly useful in relieving pyrexia and checking the return of paroxysms of intermittent fevers. The bark and the root-bark are given as a decoction or infusion. Infusion is given in doses of 25 to 75 grams twice or thrice a day. Decoction is given in doses of 150 grams between paroxysms of fever.

Stomach Disorders

Indian barberry is useful in stomach disorders. It is also effective in the treatment of cholera. It is a popular remedy for diarrhoea and dysentery in many parts of North India.

Piles

Indian barberry is useful in bleeding piles. It is given in doses of 33 to 100 centigrams with butter. A dilute solution can also be used externally for treating piles.

Menorrhagia

Indian barberry arrests any excessive blood loss during the monthly period, administered in doses of 13 to 25 centigrams.

Skin Disorders

In skin diseases, it is generally given in doses of 13 to 25 centigrams. The decoction of the bark and the root-bark is efficacious as a cleanser for ulcers and sores, as it helps cicatrization or formation of scar over the wound.

---

1. R.N. Chopra, I.C. Chopra, K.L. Handa and L.D. Kapur, Indigenous Drugs of India, 2nd edition reprint, p. 289, Academic Publishers, 1982.

Eye Disorders

The drug is highly beneficial in the treatment of eye diseases. It is mixed with butter and alum or with opium or lime juice and applied externally on eyelids to cure ophthalmia and other eye diseases. Mixed with milk, it can be used effectively as a lotion in conjunctivitis.

Method of Preparation: Root bark, roots and lower stems are boiled in water, strained and evaporated till a semi-solid mass is obtained. This is called *rasaut* which is fairly soluble in water.

Indian Mallow

Botanical Name: *Abutilan indicum.*
Indian Name: *Kanghi*

Description and Composition

Indian mallow is an erect, woody plant. It is velvety, shrubby and greyish green in colour. It grows upto one and a half metre in length. It has solitary yellow flowers which bloom in the evening. The fruits are flat-topped, with radiating points and grey, kidney-shaped seeds. The plant is covered with an aromatic oily substance. This oil coating is less pronounced in young plants than in well grown plants. Its bark, roots, leaves and seeds are all used in medicine. The plant contains an alkaloid asparagin.

Healing Power and Curative Properties

The roots and the mucilagenous bark increase the secretion and discharge of urine, besides proving to be a pulmonary sedative. The herb is laxative and tonic. It promotes libido and is useful in relieving feverishness and producing a feeling of coolness.

Fevers

The Indian mallow is valuable in fevers. Its infusion is used for this purpose.

Respiratory Disorders

A decoction of the herb can be given in bronchitis, catarrh and biliousness.

Piles

Its seeds are laxative, and very effective in curing piles, if administered in doses of 4 to 8 grams.

Skin Disorders

The drug has a soothing effect on the skin and mucous membranes. Its paste can be applied either by itself or mixed with coconut milk on the affected parts in case of abscess, carbuncle, scabies and itches. A poultice of the leaves can also be applied on boils and ulcers.

Indian mallow is useful in allaying irritation of the skin and in alleviating swelling and pain. Its decoction can be used effectively as fomentation on painful parts of the body. It can also be used as a mouthwash for toothache and tender gums.

Threadworms

The seeds are useful in killing threadworms, if the rectum of the affected child be exposed to the smoke of the powdered seeds.

Methods for Uses: The leaves should be dried in the shade and powdered for use when required. A decoction can also be extracted from the herb.

Indian Podophyllum

Botanical Name: *Podophyllum hexardrum*
Indian Name: *Papri or Banbaigan*

Description and Composition

Indian podophyllum is an erect, succulent herb with a creeping root stalk. It has flower-bearing erect branches leafy at top. The plant has toothed, purple spotted leaves, deeply divided in 3 to 5 lobes. The flowers are white or pinkish, cup-shaped and solitary. Its fruit is egg-shaped and scarlet in colour. The dried rhizomes of the plant constitute the drug.

The active principle of podophyllum is contained in the resinous mixture known as podophyllin. The other constituent of the root is podophyllotoxin. The rhizomes yield podophyllol, a sticky resin, quercetin and podophyllotoxin.

209

According to Viehoever and Mack (1938)[1], the only active crystallisable substance isolated from either podophyllum or podophyllin is podophyllotoxin. Probably, it is not the chief cathartic principle, which is still to be isolated.

Healing Power and Curative Properties

The herb podophyllum is used as a hepatic stimulant and as an agent to promote the flow of bile. It is also useful as a purgative and as a drug to correct disordered processes of nutrition and to restore the normal function of the system. It is a bitter tonic which helps induce vomiting.

Chronic Constipation

The drug is highly beneficial for treating chronic constipation and is used as a purgative. The safe single dose is 0.01 gm. Its action is slow but strong. In large doses, it can cause acute irritation and griping. It should therefore be administered either in combination with belladonna or Indian aloe.

Skin Disorders

Podophyllum is reported to be useful in many skin diseases and tumorous growths. It has acquired importance in recent years for its possible use in controlling skin cancer.

Precautions: Podophyllin greatly irritates the eyes and the mucous membranes. The resin does not affect normal skin but may be absorbed by irritated or abrased skin and helps purging. It is an effective purgative, but in toxic or over doses it produces intense enteritis or inflammation of the small intestines which may sometimes result in death.

1. Quoted from R.N. Chopra, I.C. Chopra, K.L. Handa and L.D. Kapur, Indigenous Drugs of India, p. 27, Academic Publishers, Calcutta, 1982.

Indian Sarsaparilla

Botanical Name: *Hemidesmus indicus*
Indian Name: *Magarbu or Anantmul*

Description and Composition

Indian sarsaparilla is a perennial twining or creeping herb, with a woody fragrant rootstock. It has a slender hairless stem, variable dark green leaves, greenish flowers in small compact clusters and narrow cylindrical fruits. The dried roots constitute the drug.

In the ancient Indian literature, the plant has been mentioned as an important medicine. In 1864 it was admitted in the British Pharmacopoeia.

On simple distillation with water, the roots yield a steroptency which is supposed to be a volatile acid. It also contains an essential oil. The odour of the drug is due to coumarin. The roots also contain resins, tannin and glycoside.

Healing Power and Curative Properties

The roots are a sweet tonic and exercise a soothing effect on the skin and mucous membranes. They are useful in correcting disorders due to malnutrition, purify blood, promote flow of urine and restore normal body functions.

Stomach Disorders

Indian sarsaparilla is beneficial for treating stomach disorders like dyspepsia and loss of appetite. The powder of the roots is given in doses of 1 to 6 grams with milk in these conditions. The roots ground a paste with water and mixed with pepper is useful in stomach ache and diarrhoea.

Genito-Urinary Disorders

The herb is very useful in syphilis, leucorrhoea and other genito-urinary diseases. A decoction of its roots is to be administered in 60 to 90 ml doses thrice a day. A syrup made from its roots is an effective diuretic.

Fevers

The drug is beneficial in the treatment of fevers. Its diaphoretic properties, that is, sweat inducing properties, induce copious perspiration, thereby reducing the temperature.

Inflammation

A paste of its roots is applied locally in treating swellings, rheumatic joints and boils.

Methods for Uses and Dosages: Powder of roots which are small and black should be used in tea or syrup. About 30 to 60 grams of the root powder may be used. Addition of rose petals, lotus petals, milk and honey or palm sugar to the decoction, make it a refreshing summer drink.

Other Uses

Hair Tonic: The herb contains a hair-growing hormone. A decoction of the root, used as a hair wash promotes hair growth.

Indian Senna

Botanical Name: *Cassia angustifolia*
Indian Name: *Bhumiari*

Description and Composition

Indian senna is a small bushy plant. The leaves of this plant have 5 to 8 pairs of leaflets, with awl-shaped, spreading or reflexed basal appendages. The plant has flower in racemes, that is, inflorescence on which flowers are borne, and broadly oblong and slightly curved pods.

Healing Power and Curative Properties

Indian senna is effective as a safe purgative for expelling intestinal worms.

Constipation

Senna leaves are a sure and effective purgative, even for children, weak and elderly persons. They may cause nausea and griping unless taken with aromatics like ginger, cloves, dill, fennel, coriander, orange peel or liquorice. Senna pods too can be used as a purgative but are milder and slower in action than the leaves.

Intestinal Worms

Senna can be used as an anthelmentic for killing intestinal worms.

Skin Disorders

A paste of the dried leaves made with vinegar as a base can be used for acne, eczema and pimples.

Other Diseases

Senna leaves are also effective in biliousness, gout and rheumatism, if administered in the same manner as for constipation.

Preparation and Doses: Its leaves can be given as an infusion, decoction, powder or confection. One of the best preparations is made by infusing 60 grams of the leaves and 4 grams of ginger in about half a litre of water in a covered vessel for 15 minutes. About 15 to 30 grams of this infusion should be taken with hot milk and sugar. Another method of taking the leaves is to infuse a dozen leaves in 60 ml of water overnight. The strained liquid should be taken in the morning on an empty stomach.

In case of pods, an infusion made of 4 to 12 pods in 240 ml of water can be used for adults. For children and the aged, the infusion should be made from 3 to 6 pods.

Precaution: The sennosides in senna are cathartic. Like all anthraquinones they irritate the bowel wall, stimulating evacuation. Constant use of this herb is not advised since the system can easily become dependent on it. The remedy should not be used in cases of spastic or spasmodic constipation. Similarly, it should not be given in inflammatory conditions of the alimentary canal, fever, piles and in case of excessive blood loss during menstruation.

Indian Squill

Botanical Name: *Urginea indica*
Indian Name: *Jungli piyaz*

Description and Composition

Indian squill is a bulbous plant with a smooth surface. It has egg-shaped, long, dull white or pale, thick bulbs measuring 5 to 10 cms. It has extremely narrow leaves and light brown flowers in slender long bunches. Its fruits are three-celled capsules with flat black seeds. The dry outer coats of its bulbs are removed before slicing and drying. This constitutes the drug.

Fresh squill consists of two glycosides, scillaren A which is crystalline and scillaren B which is amorphous.

Healing Power and Curative Properties

Indian squill is considered as effective as the European counterpart in therapeutic value. In small doses, the bulb is stimumlant and digestive. It is useful in removing any obstruction to secretion or excretion by opening the natural passages or pores of the body. In large doses, it is an acrid poison, inducing nausea and active movement of the bowels.

Respiratory Disorders

Indian squill promotes the removal of catarrhal matter. Clinical trials have confirmed its efficacy. It helps to remove phlegm from the bronchial tubes in asthma, bronchial catarrah and chronic bronchitis. Its juice should be administered with honey.

Dropsy

The bulb is beneficial in the treatment of dropsy. It has diuretic properties and increases the volume of urine.

Warts and Corns

For removing warts, a powder of the bulb should be applied locally on the affected areas. For corns, a poultice of the roasted bulb should be applied.

Menstrual Disorders

Indian squill is useful in promoting and regulating menstrual periods. It should be given in small doses.

Other Diseases

The herb is beneficial in the treatment of several other diseases such as rheumatism, calculus affections, chronic Bright's disease—a typical degeneration of the kidneys, leprosy, ringworm and scabies.

Jaundice Berry

Botanical Name: *Berberis vulgaris*
Indian Name: *Ambarbaris*

Description and Composition

Jaundice berry or Maider berry is an erect thorny shrub with dark brown bark and yellow wood. It has stalked, thin and egg-shaped leaves in bunches of 10, with yellow flowers and red, oblong berries.

The bark contains many active alkaloids, like berberine, oxyacanthine, and columbamine which are all antibacterial. Berberine also has antiviral properties. Tannin, resin, fat and starch are other constituents of the herb.

Healing Power and Curative Properties

The bark of its stem and root are tonic. They induces active movement of the bowels, increase the secretion and discharge of urine and reduce fever due to antibilious and antiseptic properties.

Liver Disorders

Jaundice berry is particularly useful as a bitter tonic in jaundice and other liver disorders. The pulverized bark is given several times a day in doses of quarter teaspoon. Alternatively, the fluid extract can be given in 2 or 4 gram doses.

High Blood Pressure

The herb is highly beneficial in the treatment of high blood pressure. Research has shown that it dilates the arteries thereby lowering blood pressure.

Scurvy

The leaves of the plant are antiscorbutic or anti-scurvy. A decoction of the leaves as well as the juice of the berry can be given with beneficial results in scurvy.

Fevers

The berries contain citric and malic acids useful in arresting secretion or bleeding and in promoting the flow of bile. Their juice can be given in inflammatory and malignant fevers, especially typhus and typhoid, in doses of 2 to 4 grams.

Menstrual Disorders

The herb is useful in menstrual disorders such as painful periods and excessive loss of blood. It has also been found beneficial during labour.

Precaution: This herb should not be used during pregnancy as the alkaloid berberine stimulates the uterus, and may cause abortion.

Other Uses

A Purgative: Jaundice berry acts as an effective purgative when taken in large doses of more than one fourth of a teaspoon of pulverized bark or 4 gram doses of the fluid extract.

Leadwort

Botanical Name: *Plumbago zeylanica*
Indian Name: *Chitra*

Description and Composition

Leadwort is a shrubby perennial herb with acrid roots. It grows densely upto two metres high, with 10 to 20 stems growing directly from the root. The plant has smooth leaves and tiny, bright red flowers.

The herb contains an orange yellow pigment, plumbagin, a sitosterol and a fatty alcohol. The proportion of the plumbagin varies within the limits according to the locality, growth, age, condition of the soil and the season. The older the plant and drier the soil, the greater is the quantity of active principle found in its roots.

Healing Power and Curative Properties

The root of the plant is acrid and stimulant. It is useful in inducing copious perspiration and in promoting salivation. It also strengthens the stomach and aids in its action. Its leaves are almost tasteless, have hard cellulose and are slightly mucilaginous. About 60 ml of raw juice of its leaves can be taken by itself or may be added to mixed green vegetables and lettuces to prepare gruel or cake.

Intestinal Disorders

Its leaves are useful in dyspepsia diarrhoea and piles. It increases digestive powers and stimulates appetite.

Skin Disorders

Owing to its skin irritating property the herb is used in the treatment of chronic skin diseases as well as in leucoderma and baldness. A paste made with salt and water is useful for obstinate skin diseases such as syphilitic ulcers, scabies, varicose ulcers and ringworm. Paste of the root is also used over glandular tumours and abscesses. The juice of its root, especially if fresh, is very acrid and blisters the skin.

Rheumatism

The herb is useful in the treatment of rheumatic and paralytic affections. Blended with a little bland oil such as refined coconut oil, it is applied externally over the affected parts.

Precautions: The root in large doses is narcotic and irritant. It should therefore be given only in small doses of 0.75 to 1.25 grams.

Lemon Balm

Botanical Name: *Melissa officinalis*
Indian Name: *Bililotan*

Description and Composition

Lemon balm is a perennial herb of the mint family. It grows upto 30 to 60 cm in height and lasts for two years or longer. It has a creeping root system, but is easy to keep in check. The plant has egg-shaped leaves and small white or pale pink flowers. It has a strong and agreeable odour, reminiscent of lemon, which gives it the name lemon balm. Its leaves and flowering tops constitute the drug.

The herb is said to promote longevity. Lemon balm was prescribed by the London Dispensary in the 17th century to be taken every morning to renew youthful vigour, strengthen the brain, relieve languishing nature and prevent baldness. A Welsh prince, who lived upto 108 years, attributed his longevity to regular drinking of balm tea.

The herb yields a very small quantity of essential oil. This oil comprises of citral citronellal euginol acetate, geraniol ect.

Healing Power and Curative Properties

Lemon balm is considered beneficial in strengthening the functions of stomach and promoting its action.

Nervous Disorders

Lemon balm is valuable for the brain and for strengthening memory. It prevents brain fatigue, sharpens comprehension, counteracts depression and revives the spirit. A cold infusion of the balm has a calming effect on the nerves. About 30 grams of the herb is put in half a litre of cold water and allowed to stand for 12 hours. The infusion is then strained and taken in small doses throughout the day.

Fevers

The herb is antipyretic and useful in treating fevers. Tea made from the leaves brings down the body temperature.

Other Diseases

The herb is useful in treating several other diseases. It is used to strengthen the gums and remove bad taste from the mouth. Leaves and stems are considered useful in liver and heart diseases as also in venomous insects bites.

Methods of Preservation: The plants are cut when they are in full bloom and dried in shade to preserve the natural colour.

Lemon Grass

Botanical Name: *Cymbopogon citratus*
Indian Name: *Bhustrina or Gandhatrana*

Description and Composition

Lemon grass is a perennial, aromatic, tall grass with rhizomes and densely tufted fibrous roots. It has short underground stems with ringed segments; coarse, green slightly leathery leaves in dense clusters, terminating in a long bristly point. The blades of the grass are about 90 cms long and 0.5 cm wide.

Lemon grass contains an essential oil. This oil is sherry

coloured with a pungent taste and lemon-like odour with citral as the principal constituent. The contents of this oil varies with the age of the grass. Fresh lemon grass contains an essential oil which has substantial amount of citral. Dry herb yields 0.4 per cent essential oil containing 72.3 per cent citral.

Healing Power and Curative Properties

The grass is stimulant, tonic, aromatic, antispasmodic and a mild counter-irritant. It increases secretion and discharge of urine. Oil distilled from its leaves is used for medicinal purposes.

Flatulence

Lemon grass and its oil are carminative, valuable in relieving flatulence. It is given in doses of 3 to 6 drops with sugar as an emulsion. The emulsion is prepared by mixing 3 to 6 drops of common lemon grass oil with sugar.

Digestive Disorders

Lemon grass is useful in strengthening the functions of stomach and promoting its action. It is beneficial in the treatment of indigestion. Lemon grass oil also treats spasmodic affections of the bowels, gastric irritability and cholera.

Fevers

The grass induces copious perspiration and brings down temperature. It also produces a feeling of coolness. Raw juice or decoction of the grass can also be taken.

Menstrual Disorders

An infusion of the grass, mixed with black pepper, is given in painful and difficult menstruation. Raw juice or decoction of the grass may be taken in such a condition.

Rheumatism and Other Joint Pains

The grass is used locally over rheumatic joints, lumbago and sprains. Lemon grass oil mixed with twice its bulk of coconut oil is a stimulating ointment for rheumatism, lumbago, neuralgia, sprains and other painful affections. In chronic cases, the undiluted oil may be used for better results. It can also be taken internally in the same manner as for fevers.

Ringworm

Leaves of lemon grass are useful in treating ringworm as a local application. A paste of the leaves made with buttermilk should be applied on the affected part.

Linseed

Botanical Name: *Linum usitatissimum*
Indian Name: *Alsi*

Description and Composition

Linseed is one of the most important oilseeds. It is a many-branched bushy annual plant, with erect, slender stems growing upto 30 cms high. It has alternate, stalkless leaves and blue flowers in loose clusters. The fruits are roundish, and 10-celled. Each cell contains one seed which is oval, smooth, shining and usually brown-coloured. Linseed is one of the first crops to be cultivated for its oil, bark fibre and flax.

An analysis of linseed shows it to contain moisture 6.5 per cent, protein 20.3 per cent, fat 37.1 per cent, minerals 2.4 per cent, fibre 4.8 per cent and carbohydrates 28.9 per cent per 100 grams of edible portion. Its mineral and vitamin contents are calcium, phosphorus, iron, carotene, thiamine, riboflavin and niacin. Its calorific value is 530. Linseed contains substantial amount of oil. This oil is a very valuable source of linoleic acid. It contains linoleic and linolenic acids.

Healing Power and Curative Properties

Seeds and oil of the plant are both used for their medicinal properties. The seeds increase the volume of urine.

Respiratory Disorders

The seeds are beneficial in the treatment of respiratory diseases besides being a useful remedy for colds, coughs, sore chest, throat and pulmonary complaints. Linseed tea or infusion can be given repeatedly in one glass doses. For cough and colds, the tea is given with honey. An infusion made by soaking 30 grams of the powdered seeds overnight in a glass of water can be given with lime juice in tuberculosis with beneficial results.

Genito-Urinary Disorders

The seeds are valuable in gonorrhoea, irritations of the genito-urinary organs, nephritis and cystitis, provided taken in the form of tea repititively.

Constipation

One or two teaspoons of seeds with water can treat constipation.

Chest Complaints

A loose poultice of the seeds can be applied with excellent results in chest troubles and diseases like pneumonia, bronchitis, broncho-pneumonia and pleurisy. The counter-irritant effect of the poultice can be enhanced by dusting mustard powder over it.

Linseed emulsion or tea can be made by heating a teaspoon of the powdered seeds in about 360 ml of water. The liquid is reduced to half its quantity by boiling, and can be sweetened with sugar candy or sugar. Even children can be given this tea to counteract wheezing or asthma.

Skin Disorders

A hot poultice of the seeds is a popular household remedy for skin diseases like boils, abscesses and carbuncles. Equal parts of linseed oil and lime water mixed together is an effective remedy for burns, scalds and skin diseases like eczema and herpes. Its oil is also used for removing blemishes from the face.

Methods of Preservation: The seeds are roasted over slow fire, powdered and stored for use when needed.

Marigold

Botanical Name: *Calendula officinalis*
Indian Name: *Saldbargh or Zergul*

Description and Composition

Marigold is a hairy annual herb, growing to about 50 cms high. The lower leaves of the plant are strapshaped and the base of the upper leaves surround the stem. The plant has large, solitary and stout flower heads; flat and spreading flowers of the outer whorl, with colour varying from light yellow to deep orange. The fruits are curved, with the lower part having sharp point and upper parts crested and slightly beaked.

The main constituents of the herb are carotenoids, resin,

essential oil, flavonoids, sterol, saponins and mucilage.

Healing Power and Curative Properties

Marigold is a bitter tonic. It induces copious perspiration and is useful in killing intestinal worms.

Digestive Disorders

The herb stimulates the flow of bile, and is a beneficial remedy in the treatment of gastritis, gastric or duodenal ulcers.

Scrofula

The leaves are useful in treating scrofula or tuberculosis of the lymphatic glands in children, especially in the neck. As a remedy the leaves should be taken as a vegetable.

Circulatory Disorders

It is beneficial in the treatment of certain circulatory disorders. A compress of the herb can be applied beneficially in the treatment of varicose veins and chilblains, which is an inflamed condition of the skin of the hands, feet and sometimes ears and nose caused by poor circulation and cold weather.

Skin Disorders

Marigold belongs to the same family as arnica and has umpteem wound-healing properties. It is antiseptic and anti-bacterial. A compress or poultice of the flowers forms an excellent first aid for burns, scalds, stings and impetigo, a highly contagious bacterial skin infection. The juice of the leaves can be applied beneficially over warts. The sap from the stem is useful for warts, corns and callouses.

Marigold flowers are an excellent remedy for inflamed or ulcerated conditions of the skin when used externally, as in varicose ulcers.

Conjunctivitis

A cold infusion of the herb, used as an eyewash, gives relief in conjunctivitis. A lotion of the flowers is also a useful wash for inflamed and sore eyes.

Marjoram

Botanical Name: *Origanum majorana*
Indian Name: *Marwa*

Description and Composition

Marjoram or sweet marjoram is an aromatic herb of the mint family which grows upto 30 to 60 cm high. Though perennial, it is treated as an annual herb under cultivation. It has small leaves hairy on either sides; tiny green, white flowers, forming small branched heads, which look like knots.

The dried leaves of marjoram with or without flowering tops in small proportions, constitute the herb. It has a fragrant, spicy, slightly sharp, bitter and camphoraceous flavour. The colour of the dried herb is light green with a greyish tint.

Fractional distillation of the leaves and flowering heads yield a volatile oil, known as oil of sweet marjoram. However, the yield from the fresh herb is less than that from the dried herb. The oil is colourless or pale yellow to yellow-green, with a persistent odour reminiscent of nutmeg and mint.

Healing Power and Curative Properties

Sweet majoram is stimulant and tonic. Its flowers and seeds are useful in arresting secretion or bleeding.

Common Cold

The warmth accumulated by the herb from the sun helps to clear bad colds. Tea made from majoram has the ability to stimulate the sweat glands. It helps to moisten taut, dry skin during influenza, if taken in small quantities.

Asthma

The herb helps expel and loosen phlegm of the mucous membranes of the nasal and bronchial passages.

Women's Ailments

Marjoram is useful in promoting and regulating menstruation if taken in the form of an infusion. Such an infusion helps in promoting the secretion and flow of milk in nursing mothers.

Digestive Disorders

Marjoram is beneficial in the treatment of digestive

disorders. It expels gas from the stomach. Hot fomentations of the dried leaves and tops applied in bags is helpful in colic. The oil of marjoram can be used beneficially as hot fomentation in acute diarrhoea.

Skin Disorders

The oil of marjoram is useful in skin disorders and it can be applied externally in case of sprains, bruises, stiff and paralytic limbs. It also allays toothache.

Parslane

Botanical Name: *Portulaca oleracea*
Indian Name: *Kulfa*

Description and Composition

Parslane is a small, smooth fleshy annual herb and a popular green leafy vegetable. It grows upto 30 cms in height. It has very few branches and the stem is feeble, smooth, shiny and light pink in colour. The leaves are simple, thick, smooth and succulent. Its has yellow flowers and small fruits containing numerous black seeds.

An analysis of parslane shows it to consist of moisture 90.5 per cent, protein 2.4 per cent, fat 0.6 per cent, minerals 2.3 per cent, fibre 1.3 per cent and carbohydrates 2.9 per cent per 100 grams. Its mineral and vitamin contents are calcium, phosphorus, iron, carotene, thiamine, riboflavin, niacin and vitamin C. Its calorific value is 27.

Healing Power and Curative Properties

The leaves are mildly salty, sour and contain mucilage. They are refrigerant and produce a feeling of coolness. They are useful in correcting disorders due to malnutrition. Its seeds exercise a soothing effect on the skin and mucous membranes. They are also useful in arresting bleeding, increasing the secretion as well as the discharge of urine.

Urinary Disorders

The herb is a valuable diet in dysuria, which is marked by pain or difficulty in passing urine. The leaves are also useful in this disorder. A teaspoon of the infusion is given twice a day. Its seeds are useful in treating scanty urination due to excessive sweating. A teaspoon of emulsion of the seeds prepared by mixing a teaspoon of the seeds in a glass of tender coconut water and administered thrice daily can cure such disorders. It also reduces the burning sensation of cystitis.

Diarrhoea and Dysentery

In diarrhoea and dysentery, the seeds relieve griping pains, tenesmus which is the ineffectual straining to relieve the bowels and other painful effects of dysentery and mucuous diarrhoea. They should preferably be given in combination with other drugs or herbs like fenugreek leaves, mint juice and powdered mango seeds.

Diabetes

A teaspoon of its seed taken everyday with water for three to four months can increase the body's own insulin and help in curing diabetes.

Expectorating Blood

Its leaves are beneficial in the treatment of mild type of blood expectoration—that is bleeding from the mouth, nose and rectum. The juice from its leaves, mixed with a teaspoon of fresh lime juice and honey, is taken thrice daily.

Skin Disorders

A poultice of the leaves can be applied with beneficial results to burns, scalds and many other skin diseases like boils, ulcers, wounds and carbuncles. It can also be applied as a coolant in erysipelas, a streptococcal infection of the skin. Its leaves are useful in allaying irritations of the skin and in reducing swelling and pain.

Prickly Heat and Burning Sensation

Parslane is commonly used as a medicine to cool the body during summer. The juice of its stem can be applied with gratifying results to prickly heat and to allay heat and burning of hands and feet. The paste of its leaves can also be used similarly. A poultice of the leaves can be applied to the temples as an emollient to allay pain.

Pergularia

Botanical Name: *Pergularia extensa*
Indian Name: *Uttran or Sadorani*

Description and Composition

Pergularia is a perennial, small, twining herb. It has hairy stems with milky juice and broad, egg-shaped leaves. It has greenish yellow or dull white, small flowers in tiny clusters and fruits reflexed in pairs, covered with spinous outgrowths. The entire plant constitutes the drug and is used as medicine.

It contains a bitter resin, two bitter principles and a glucoside possessing physiological action similar to pituitrin and several sterols.

Healing Power and Curative Properties

Pergularia is pungent, antibilious and laxative. It is useful in relieving fever and inducing vomiting. The active principles of pergularia resemble pituitrin in their action.

Respiratory Disorders

Pergularia promotes the removal of catarrhal matter and phlegm from the bronchial tubes. It is highly beneficial in the treatment of asthma. The juice from the leaves is used as an expectorant in catarrhal diseases. A decoction of its leaves is given in cough as an expectorant.

Intestinal Worms

The drug possesses anthelmintic properties and finds its use in removing intestinal worms. About 24 grams of the leaves fried in *ghee* should be taken for a few days.

Piles

The herb is beneficial in the treatment of bleeding piles. It should be used in the same manner as for intestinal worms.

Rheumatism

Pergularia forms a constituent of a preparation used in rheumatism. The leaf juice can be given mixed with the juice of fresh ginger in the treatment. The root bark is also useful in the treatment of rheumatism. It should be given in 4 to 8 gram doses with milk. The bark, mixed with cow's milk, can be used beneficially as a purgative in rheumatic complaints.

Women's Disorders

The drug is a useful uterine tonic. It is beneficial in excessive uterine bleeding. The drug forms a constituent of a preparation given in amenorrhoea or abnormal suppression of menses.

Infantile Diarrhoea

The juice of its leaves can be given to treat diarrhoea among children.

Stranguary

The drug has diuretic properties. It is valuable in stranguary, that is, discharge of urine in droplets accompanied by pain.

Skin Disorders

The herb is beneficial in the treatment of several skin disorders. A mixture of the leaf juice and slaked lime can be applied to rheumatic swellings, hard tumours and cysts. A poultice of the leaves can be applied to carbuncles with beneficial effect.

Picrorhiza

Botanical Name: *Picrorhiza kurroa*
Indian Name: *Kutki or Kuru*

Description and Composition

Picrorhiza is a small, hairy perennial herb with woody rhizomes. It has small white or pale bluish purple flowers in cylindric spikes. The dried rhizomes of the plant constitute the drug. Its trade name picrorhiza is based on its scientific name.

The drug contains bitter glucoside kutkin, a non bitter product kurrin, vanillic acid, an alcohol kutkiol, a sterol kutikisterol and an odorous principle, sesquiterpene. The herb is used extensively in conditions in which the drugs with taste are considered significant. The drug is a recognised substitute for the European gentian in Indian Pharmaceutical Codex 1952.

Healing Power and Curative Properties

The herb is considered in the indigenous medicine to be a valuable bitter tonic, almost as efficacious as Indian gentian, botanically known as *gentian kurroo (nilkenta)*. It cures periodic attacks like hysteria, epilepsy and convulsion and promotes the secretion of bile. It has antibiotic properties.

Cirrhosis of Liver

Picrorhiza is a choice drug for cirrhosis of the liver among adults in *Ayurveda*. Its root is given in powdered form. A teaspoon of the powder, mixed with an equal amount of honey, is administered thrice daily. In case of attendant constipation, the dose should be doubled and taken with a cup of warm water three to four times a day. It stimulates the liver to produce more bile, the secretion of which relieves congestion of the liver and the tissues which start functioning again.

Jaundice

Picrorhiza is one of the two major drugs considered beneficial in *Ayurveda* for the treatment of jaundice, the other drug being turpeth *(nisoth)*. One or two teaspoons of the powder of the two drugs should be administered with hot water twice daily.

Indigestion

Picrorhiza is beneficial in the treatment of dyspepsia. It strengthens the stomach and promotes its action, while improving appetite and stimulating the secretion of gastric juices.

Constipation

The herb is very useful in constipation. It induces active movement of the bowels and serves as a mild purgative.

Ascites

Picrorhiza is beneficial in the treatment of ascites, a disease characterised by the accumulation of fluid in the peritoneal cavity of the abdomen. About 50 grams of the herb is boiled in 200 ml of water till three-fourths of the water has evaporated. This decoction if taken by the patient for 21 days regularly, with fresh decoction each day can induce 4 to 5 motions on an average, leading to reduction of girth of his/her abnormal belly.

Saffron

Botanical Name: *Crocus sativus*
Indian Name: *Kesar or Zaafaran*

Description and Composition

Saffron is a plant resembling onion, 45 cms high. Commercial saffron consists of the dried stigma and tops of the styles of the flowers. It is one of the world's costliest herbs. Saffron is more popular in the Tibbi than in the Ayurvedic medicine.

Saffron contains an essential oil which consists of terpenes, terpene alcohols and esters. Its other constituents are crocin and picrocrocin.

Healing Power and Curative Properties

Saffron is largely used in indigenous medicine across India. It enjoys a great reputation as a drug which strengthens the functioning of stomach and promotes its action. The drug also counteracts spasmodic disorders, that is, sustained involuntary muscle contraction. It is a stimulant and promotes libido.

Digestive Disorders

Saffron is beneficial in the treatment of several digestive disorders, especially flatulent colic.

Women's Ailments

The herb is useful in promoting and regulating menstrual periods. It soothes lumbar pains which accompany menstruation. Saffron is also beneficial in the treatment of other ailments concerning women such as leucorrhoea and hysteria. Pessaries of saffron are used in painful conditions of the uterus.

Skin Disorders

Saffron is useful in treating skin disorders. A paste of the herb can be used as a dressing for bruises and superficial sores.

Precautions: The drug should not be taken in large doses by pregnant women as it may cause abortion.

Snake Gourd

Botanical Name: *Trichosanthes anguina*
Indian Name: *Chachinga*

Description and Composition

Snake gourd is a climbing herb with tendrils divided into three parts. It has hairy, angular or 5 to 7 lobed leaves which emit a foetid odour when bruised. It has white male and female flowers and cylindrical, slender, tapering fruits with a waxy surface. Its fruits are orange in colour when ripe, and pulpy red at maturity.

An analysis of snake gourd shows it to consist of substantial amount of moisture and little protein, fat, fibre and carbohydrate. Its mineral and vitamin contents are calcium, phosphorus, iron, substantial amount of carotene, little thiamine, riboflavin and niacin. Its calorific value is 18.

Healing Power and Curative Properties

The plant is a cardiac tonic and antifebrile, that is, counteracts feverishness. It is useful in restoring the disordered processes of nutrition. It creates a cooling effect in the body. Being a low-calorie food, diabetics can safely include it to reduce weight while getting enough nutrition. Its leaves are used in indigenous medicine in India.

Heart Disorders

The juice of the fresh leaves is useful in heart disorders like palpitation and pain in the heart on physical exertion. It should be taken in doses of 1 to 2 tablespoons thrice daily.

Jaundice

Infusion of the leaves is beneficial in the treatment of jaundice, if given in 30 to 60 gram doses with a decoction of coriander seeds thrice daily.

Fevers

A decoction of snake gourd is useful in bilious fevers, as a febrifuge or thirst reliever and laxative. Its efficacy increases provided it is given with *chiratta* and honey. In obstinate cases of fevers, a combined infusion of this plant and coriander is more beneficial. About 30 grams of each should be infused in water overnight. The strained liquid should be given in two doses

230

the next day. A decoction of the leaves with the addition of coriander is also useful in bilious fever. The leaf juice is used to induce vomiting. The latter is also applied locally as a liniment in cases of liver congestion. In remittent fevers, it is applied over the whole body.

Alopecia

The leaf juice is beneficial in the treatment of alopecia, a disease of the scalp resulting in complete or partial baldness.

Precaution: The ripe fruit and its seeds are laxative and may cause indigestion, and should not be consumed as food.

Other Uses

Purgative: Its root serves as purgative and tonic. Whereas its juice is a strong purgative, an infusion of the dried fruit is a mild purgative. It also aids digestion. Its leaves are useful as an emetic and purgative in children suffering from constipation. A teaspoon of the fresh juice can be given early in the morning for the ailing children.

The immature fruits can be boiled and eaten as a vegetable.

Tenner's Cassia

Botanical Name: *Cassia auriculata*
Indian Name: *Tarwar*

Description and Composition

Tenner's cassia is a well-known perennial shrub which grows upto 30 to 60 cms in height. It has a round, hard and strong stem, brown in colour, with numerous branches. It has compound, stipulate leaves, yellowish green in colour and large yellow flowers. There are 7 to 10 seeds in each of its fruits.The plant is called tenners cassia as the bark is one of the most valuable of Indian tans containing tannin.

Healing Power and Curative Properties

The bark of the plant is useful in arresting secretion or bleeding. The leaves are tonic. They relieve feverishness and produce a feeling of coolness. They also restore the disordered processes of nutrition. Its leaves and petals are both mildly

231

astringent in taste. The leaves contain a small quantity of mucilage, though they are completely non-poisonous, the taste and smell are unpalatable. An infusion of the leaves makes a cooling drink. Its seeds also have a cooling effect.

Diabetes

Tenner's cassia is useful in diabetes. A decoction of the whole plant or buds can be used to treat this disease. The powder of the herb, mixed with honey, is equally efficacious in such a case. Its seeds can be used in the similar manner as flowers.

Conjunctivitis

Finely powdered, decorticated seeds should be used as a dusting powder in the treatment of conjunctivitis.

Sore Throat

The bark of the plant has astringent properties and is useful as a gargle in case of sore throat.

Menstruation

The herb is useful in regulating the menstrual cycle. The flowers and flower buds can be used beneficially as pessaries to check excessive menstrual flow.

Ophthalmia

The seeds find their application in purulent ophthalmia ---that is, inflammation of the eye or conjunctiva. They should be finely powdered and blown into the affected eyes. An ointment prepared from them and oil can be applied to the affected eye with confidence.

Wormwood

Botanical Name: *Artemisia absinthum*
Indian Name: *Afsanthin*

Description and Composition

Wormwood is an aromatic, bitter, hairy perennial herb. It has erect, angular and ribbed stems, 30 to 90 cms high. It has egg-shaped leaves, 2.5 to 5.0 cm long which are hairy on both sides and unequally cut into segments. It also has numerous,

minute yellow drooping flower heads and sn
seeded fruit.

The Latin name of the herb comes from the
Artemis, who took care of women during childbirth
to bring on periods and could be used externally as a c
during labour to speed up birth and afterwards, internall
externally to expel the placenta.

The active principles of Indian wormwood consists of volatile
oil which has an odour resembling cajuput oil and camphor,
santonin and an allied body artemisin.

Healing Power and Curative Properties

The whole herb is used medicinally, but its leaves are
preferred. The fresh plant is considered more efficacious than
a dry one. The herb is a tonic, useful in strengthening the
functioning of stomach and promoting its action. It stimulates
appetite, the digestive juices, peristalsis or movement of the
bowels, the liver and gall bladder. True to its name, it also expels
intestinal worms, especially round and thread-worms.

Intestinal Worms

Wormwood had been used by ancient Greek, Roman, Arab
and Persian physicians to expel intestinal worms. The flowering
tops have been, and are still, used in the Tibbi medicine in India
as a drug to kill intestinal worms. They are usually powdered
and administered in 8 to 16 gram doses for roundworms and
tapeworms.

The oil distilled from the plant also possesses the property
to kill worms. Mixed with eight times its weight of olive oil, it can
be given in doses of 50 to 100 grams. An infusion of the herb
can be given as an enema for killing worms in the rectum.

Bilious Disorders

The herb is beneficial in the treatment of bilious melancholia
besides dispersing the yellow bile of jaundice from the skin. An
infusion of the herb or its powder can be given in small doses.

Skin Disorders

Wormwood helps disperse or absorb a tumour or any other
coagulated fluid in case of skin diseases. It also acts as an
antiseptic and cleanser. It can be pickled in vinegar and applied
with beneficial results to sprains and bruises.

useful in several other diseases such as
digestive system, nocturnal pollutions or
sex act, involuntarily, during sleep without
emia, wasting diseases and general debility.
small doses of 0.75 to 1.25 decigrams in
essential oil of the herb is used as a cardiac
imulant.

The drug should be avoided during pregnancy
ed, should be taken only for short periods.

Valerian

Botanical Name: *Valeriana officinalis*
Indian Name: *Jalakan*

Description and Composition

Valerian is a perennial herb which grows upto 1 metre in height. Its rootstock is thicker than the stem, producing suckers or shoots rising from the ground. The stems are furrowed, hairy below and smooth above, whereas its lower leaves are long compared to the smaller upper leaves. The plant has small, white flowers in small clusters and small and smooth fruit. The rhizomes and roots of the plant constitute the drug.

According to some authorities, the name valerian is from the Latin word Valere meaning to be in health, while others believe that it takes its name from an ancient physician, Valerius, who first employed the herb in medicine.[1]

The herb contains valerianic, formic and acetic acids, in addition to an essential oil, resin, starch, a glucoside and two alkaloids---chatrine and valerianine.

Healing Power and Curative Properties

The leaves should be collected in autumn and dried slowly. The antispasmodic and stimulant properties of this plant are well

---

1. Richard Lucas, *The Magic of Herbs in Daily Living*, p. 163, Parker Publishing Company, New York, 1972.

known in indigenous medicine and have been described in the books of Ayurvedic medicine.

Nervous Disorders

Valerian is a traditional remedy for functional disturbances of the nervous system. It was perhaps the earliest treatment of neurosis, accompanied by physical diseases with mental symptoms or social maladjustment, especially in interpersonal relationships.

The herb is particularly useful in treating cases of hysteria, restless and irritable conditions. The drug exercises deppressant action on the overall central nervous system. It has gained importance in recent years owing to its beneficial effects in epilepsy. It is also considered useful in chorea, a condition marked by incessant involuntary jerks.

Insomnia

The herb is useful in treating insomnia. It reduces excitement, irritation and pain. The fresh juice of the plant can be used as a narcotic to induce sleep.

Methods for Uses and Dosages: The juice of the fresh rhizomes and roots is considered more effective in the treatment of nervous disorders as its medicinal properties get reduced on drying. An infusion of valerian is prepared by infusing 30 grams of the herb in half a litre of boiling water. The latter should be taken in small quantities three or four times daily.

Zizyphus

Botanical Name: *Zizyphus jujuba*
Indian Name: *Ber*

Description and Composition

Zizyphus is one of the most hardy fruit trees. It is a small thorny evergreen tree, with vine-like branches and dark green leaves. It has egg-shaped fruit of orange or brown in colour, with edible acid pulp and hard central stone.

The fruit has two varieties—the wild one, called *jharberi*, is small and round, while the cultivated fruit is oval, fleshy and bigger in size. It is sweeter compared to the smaller kind.

An analysis of zizyphus shows it to consist of moisture 81.6

per cent, protein 0.8 per cent, fat 0.3 per cent, minerals 0.3 per cent, and carbohydrates 17.0 per cent per 100 grams. Its mineral and vitamin contents are calcium, phosphorus, iron, carotene, thiamine, riboflavin, niacin and vitamin C. Its calorific value is 74. Both the varieties of the fruit contain zizyphic acid and tannins.

Healing Power and Curative Properties

The bark is useful in arresting secretion or bleeding. The fruit purifies the blood and aids digestion.

Mental Retardation

Zizyphus is beneficial in the treatment of mental retardation. A handful of the dry fruit is boiled in half a litre of water till it is reduced to half. Sugar or honey can be added to taste and given daily at night before retiring. It increases the functioning of the brain by releasing more glutamic acid into the bloodstream.

Colds and Influenza

Zizyphus is useful in preventing frequent attacks of colds and influenza. A teaspoon of the fresh juice of the fruit can be taken with a pinch of pepper once daily for preventing colds.

Stomach Disorders

The bark can be used for treating diarrhoea, dysentery and colic. The infusion of the inner covering of the bark is used as a purgative in constipation.

Piles

Fresh baked leaves are useful in piles. The leaves are baked by placing them over the covered mouth of a vessel with water boiling. The leaves are covered with another plate to prevent steam from escaping. Those baked leaves are pounded with some castor oil. This warm poultice can be applied over the piles. The process should be repeated twice daily for a week.

Mouth Disorders

Infusion of the fresh and tender leaves, mixed with salt is a useful gargle for sore throat, relaxed uvula, inflammation of the mouth, bleeding from gums and cracked tongue due to excessive consumption of sour fruits.

Skin Disorders

A paste of the leaves and twigs can be applied with excellent results over boils, carbuncles and abcesses to promote suppuration. It can also be applied beneficially over painful boils and styes. This paste, mixed with a teaspoon of lime juice can be applied as a poultice in the treatment of scorpion sting. Infusion of its leaves can be applied as a lotion to wash the wounds and other ulcers.

Conjunctivitis

The leaves are valuable in treating conjunctivitis. An infusion of the leaves should be used as an eye lotion.

Hair Disorders

The paste of its leaves applied over the scalp and hair can keep them clean and prevents scalp diseases. It also lengthens the hair besides darkening them.

Bibliography

1. Satyavati G.V. and Gupta Ashok K., *Medicinal Plants of India*, I.C.M.R, 1987, New Delhi.
2. Chopra R.N., Nayar S.L. and Chopra I.C., *Glossary of Indian Medicinal Plants*, C.S.I.R, 1956, New Delhi.
3. Chopra R.N., Chopra I.C., Handa, K.L and Kapur L.D., *Indigenous Drugs of India*, Academic Publishers, 1982, Calcutta.
4. Jain S.K., *Medicinal Plants*, National Book Trust, 5th edition 1985, New Delhi.
5. Dastur J.F., *Medicinal Plants of India and Pakistan*, D.B. Taraporevala Sons & Co. P. Ltd., Reprinted 1985, Bombay.
6. Aman, *Medicinal Secrets of your Food*, Indo-American Hospital, N.R. Mohalla, 1985, Mysore.
7. Agarwal V.S.[1] and Ghosh Barin, *Drug Plants of India: Root Drugs*. Kalyani Publishers, 1985, New Delhi, Ludhiana.
8. Pruthi J.S, *Spices and Condiments*., National Book Trust, 3rd edition 1987, New Delhi.
9. Ramaswami Pillai N, *Herbal Foods*. Nature Cure Publishing House, 2nd edition 1985, Pudukkottai.
10. Abdul Hamed Saheb H., *The Complete Book of Home Remedies*, Orient Paperbacks, 1982, Delhi.
11. Verma Ganpati Singh, *Miracles of Indian Herbs*, Rasayan Pharmacy, 3rd reprint 1982, New Delhi.
12. Khanna Girija, *Herbal Remedies*. Tarang Paperbacks, 4th edition 1986, New Delhi.
13. Hemphill Rosemary, *Herbs for all Seasons*, Penguin Books, 1975.
14. Lucas Richard, *The Magic of Herbs in Daily Living*, Parker Publishing Company, 1972, New York.
15. Mabey Richard, McIntyre Michael, Michael Pamela and Stevers John, *The Complete New Herbal Elm Tree Books*, 1988, London.
16. Ross Alison, *Herbal Teas for Health and Healing*, Thorsons Publishing Group, 3rd impression Novemeber 1986 Wellingborough.
17. Murthy Anjneya N. and Pandey D.P., *Ayurvedic Cure for Common Diseases*, Orient Paperbacks, 2nd edition 1983, Delhi.
18. Singh R.N. and Roy Susanta K., *The Bael Cultivation and Processing*, I.C.A.R., 1984, New Delhi.
19. Gopalan C. Rama Sastri B.V. and Balasubramanian S.C., *Nutritive Value of Indian Foods*, I.C.M.R., 1980, Hyderabad.
20. Saha N.N., *Herbal Remedies*, Universal Pub., 1987, New Delhi.

Health Care in
Orient Paperbacks

Herbal Remedies and Home Comforts

Jill Nice

Rs. 80.00

More and more people are curing their illnesses with the herbal treatments and natural preventatives that have been effectively used for thousands of years. In this fascinating book, Jill Nice, a well-respected authority on preparing herbal medicines, has compiled a huge compendium of tried and tested remedies and common-sense advice.

This is a quick and easy reference book for using safe, drug-free remedies to cure a wide range of ailments — from aches and pains to infectious diseases, from insect bites and acne to indigestion. All the remedies are easy to prepare using readily available ingredients.

But don't save *Herbal Remedies and Home Comforts* until illness strikes. It also suggests preventative measures and recommends herbals to ward off illness, as well as giving instructions for making delightful herbal preparations that will scent and purify the home to ensure a healthy atmosphere.

Available at all bookshops or by VPP

ORIENT
PAPERBACKS

Madarsa Rd, Kashmere Gate
Delhi - 110 006. India